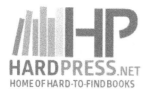

HARDPRESS.NET
HOME OF HARD-TO-FIND BOOKS

Observations on the Nature and Cure of Dropsies
by John Blackall

Address:
HardPress
8345 NW 66TH ST #2561
MIAMI FL 33166-2626
USA
Email: info@hardpress.net

TRAVELS IN AFRICA,

IN OCTAVO, WITH TWO MAPS, PRICE FOURTEEN SHILLINGS.

AN ACCOUNT

OF

TIMBUCTOO AND HOUSA,

TERRITORIES IN THE

INTERIOR OF AFRICA,

BY EL HAGE ABD SALAM SHABEENY,

A Native of Morocco,

WHO PERSONALLY VISITED AND RESIDED AS A MERCHANT IN THOSE INTERESTING COUNTRIES.

WITH NOTES, CRITICAL AND EXPLANATORY.

To which is added,

LETTERS,

DESCRIPTIVE OF VARIOUS JOURNIES THROUGH WEST AND SOUTH BARBARY,

AND

ACROSS THE MOUNTAINS OF ATLAS;

Also Fragments and Anecdotes,

AND

SPECIMENS OF THE ARABIC EPISTOLARY STYLE, &c. &c.

BY

JAMES GREY JACKSON, Esq.

RESIDENT UPWARDS OF SIXTEEN YEARS, IN THOSE COUNTRIES, AS CONSUL AND MERCHANT.

" Mr. Jackson having resided sixteen years in West and South Barbary, we may naturally give him credit for a perfect knowledge both of the language and manners of the people."

[*Turn over.*

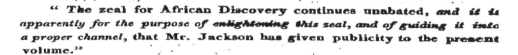

" The zeal for African Discovery continues unabated, *and it is apparently for the purpose of enlightening this zeal, and of guiding it into a proper channel*, that Mr. Jackson has given publicity to the present volume."

" In reasoning on the Geography of Africa, Mr. Jackson is not deficient in acuteness, and his thorough knowledge of the native language and manners, enables him to enter with advantage into the arena of African Geography, and occasionally to strike out unexpected lights from the analogy of African names and places. *In this respect he possesses a singular advantage over every other traveller;* his work contains various interesting sketches of a country little known, and curious interesting details of the Arab manners. We have derived both instruction and amusement from its perusal."

Edinburgh Monthly Review, Oct. 1820.

" How exceedingly interesting this work is; we shall not stop to impress, but at once proceed to our task with feelings of great pleasure and pride, at being the first to lay such remarkable communications before the public."

" Mr. Jackson has laid us under a deep obligation by his notes and intelligence concerning this third portion of the Old World; the work is replete with matter *important in African Geography*, independent of the accounts of that particular region, in the attempt to reach which, Park, and others of our enterprising countrymen perished. A long residence in the country has stored the Author's mind with a fund of interesting intelligence. The charm of variety in *this volume* is undoubtedly great, and when thrown over matter intrinsically good, he must be a sour critic indeed who can resist being highly pleased with Mr. Jackson's various and intelligent volume. The readers of this Work will find in it a great variety of interesting information respecting Africa, its geography, language, customs, &c. &c.

Literary Gazette, No. 171, pages 273, 387, 612, and 629.

PRINTED FOR LONGMAN, HURST, REES, ORME, AND BROWN, LONDON.

April, 1821.

MEDICAL WORKS
Recently published by
LONGMAN, HURST, REES, ORME, AND BROWN, LONDON.

MR. ABERNETHY.

The SURGICAL and PHYSIOLOGI-CAL WORKS of JOHN ABERNETHY, F.R.S.&c. complete in 3 vols. 8vo. Price 2l. 3s. 6d. Bds. consisting of—Part I. On the Constitutional Origin, Treatment of Local Diseases, and on Aneurisms, 8s.—Part II. On Diseases resembling Syphilis, and on Diseases of the Urethra, 6s.—Part III. On Injuries of the Head, and Miscellaneous Subjects, 7s.—Part IV. On Lumber Abscesses and Tumours, 6s.—An Inquiry into the Probability and Rationality of Mr. Hunter's Theory of Life, 4s. 6d.; an Introductory Lecture for the Year 1815, exhibiting some of Mr. Hunter's Opinions respecting Diseases, 2s. PHYSIOLOGICAL LECTURES, exhibiting a general View of Mr. Hunter's Physiology, and of his Researches in Comparative Anatomy, delivered before the Royal College of Physicians, in the Year 1817, 8s.; and the HUNTERIAN ORATION for the Year 1819, 2s. 6d.

DR. BATEMAN.

REPORTS on the DISEASES of LONDON, and the State of the Weather, from 1804 to 1816, including Practical Remarks on the Causes and Treatment of the former. By THOS. BATEMAN, M.D. F.L.S. &c. late Physician to the Public Dispensary and consulting Physician to the Fever Institution in London. In 8vo. 9s. Bds.

A SUCCINCT ACCOUNT of the CONTAGIOUS FEVER of this Country, as exemplified in the Epidemic now prevailing in London, with the appropriate Method of Treatment, as practised in the House of Recovery, and pointing out the Means of Prevention. By THOMAS BATEMAN, M.D. 2nd Edit. 8vo. Price 6s. Bds.

DELINEATIONS of the CUTANEOUS DISEASES, comprised in the Classification of the late Dr. Willan; including the greater part of the Engravings of that Author, in an improved State, and completing the Series as intended to have been finished by him. By T. BATEMAN, M. D. In 1 vol. 4to. with upwards of 70 coloured plates. Price 12l. 12s. boards.

The Series of New Engravings, representing those Diseases which should have been figured in the subsequent parts of Dr. Willan's unfinished Work, may be had by the possessors of that Work, separate. Price 7l. Boards.

A PRACTICAL SYNOPSIS of CUTANEOUS DISEASES, according to the Arrangement of Dr. WILLAN, exhibiting a concise View of the Diagnostic Symptoms, and the Method of Treatment. By THOMAS BATEMAN, M. D. In 8vo. (illustrated by a coloured Plate of the Eight Orders), the Fifth Edition. 12s. Bds.

MR. BRODIE.

PATHOLOGICAL and SURGICAL OBSERVATIONS on DISEASES of the JOINTS. By B. C. BRODIE, F. R. S. Assistant Surgeon to St. George's Hospital, and Lecturer on Surgery. In 1 Vol. 8vo. illustrated by Plates. Price 16s. Bds.

MR. CHARLES BELL.

The ANATOMY of the HUMAN BODY, containing the Anatomy of the Bones, Muscles, Joints, Heart, and Arteries. By JOHN BELL, Surgeon. And that of the Brain and Nerves, the Organs of the Senses, and the Viscera. By CHARLES BELL, Surgeon. In 3 vols. 8vo. (with numerous Engravings). price 2l. 12s. 6d. Boards. The Fourth Edition.

ILLUSTRATIONS of the Great OPERATIONS of SURGERY, TREPHINE, HERNIA, AMPUTATION, ANEURISM, and LITHOTOMY. By CHARLES BELL. In large 4to. with Twenty Plates, price 3l. 15s. plain, or 5l. 5s. coloured impressions.

By the same Author,

A SYSTEM of OPERATIVE SURGERY, founded on the Basis of Anatomy. In 2 vols. 8vo. Price 1l. 18s. Bds. The 2d Edit. (illustrated with upwards of 100 Engravings). This Edition includes a Dissertation on Gunshot Wounds, by the same Author.

The ANATOMY of the BRAIN; explained in a Series of Engravings, beautifully coloured, with a Dissertation on the Communication between the Ventricles of the Brain. In royal 4to. Price 2l. 2s. in Boards.

A SERIES of ENGRAVINGS, explaining the Course of the Nerves. New Edition. Price 1l. 1s. in Boards.

A DISSERTATION on GUN-SHOT WOUNDS. In royal 8vo. illustrated by 17 Engravings, Price 10s. 6d. in Boards. Uniform with the First Edition of the Operative Surgery.

ENGRAVINGS of the ARTERIES, illustrating the Second Volume of the Anatomy of the Human Body, by JOHN BELL, Surgeon; and serving as an Introduction to the Surgery of the Arteries, by CHARLES BELL, Surgeon. Superbly printed in Imperial 8vo. The Third Edition. Price 15s. in Boards; or with Plates, finely coloured, Price 1l. 1s. Boards.

ENGRAVINGS from SPECIMENS of MORBID PARTS, preserved in Mr Charles Bell's Collection now in Windmill Street, and selected from the Divisions inscribed Urethra, Vesica, Ren, Morbosa et Læsa. Fasciculus I. Price 1l. 16s. sewed.

A SYSTEM of DISSECTIONS; explaining the Anatomy of the Human Body; and pointing out to the Student the Objects most worthy his Attention, during a Course of Dissections. The 3d Edit. 2 vols. foolscap. Price 12s. Bds.

MR. JOHN BELL.

The PRINCIPLES of SURGERY, as they relate to Wounds, Ulcers, and Fistulas; Aneurism and Wounded Arteries; Fractures of the Limbs; and the Duties of the Military and Hospital Surgeon.

By JOHN BELL, Surgeon.

In 3 large vols. royal 4to. illustrated by upwards of 160 Engravings, many of them accurately coloured from Nature. Price 7*l.* 4*s.* Boards.

———————— Volume the Second, may be had separate. Price 3*l.* 12*s.* bds.

———————— Volume the Third, separate. Price 1*l.* 4*s.* Bds.

ENGRAVINGS of the BONES, MUSCLES, and JOINTS, illustrating the First Volume of the Anatomy of the Human Body.

By JOHN BELL, Surgeon. In 4to. with about 200 Pages of Explanatory Letter press. The Third Edition. Price 1*l.* 11*s.* 6*d.* in Boards.

DR. BLACKALL.

OBSERVATIONS on the NATURE and CURE of DROPSIES.

By JOHN BLACKALL, M. D. Physician of the Devon and Exeter Hospital, and of the Lunatic Asylum, near Exeter.

In 8vo. the Third Edition, Price 10*s.* 6*d.* Boards.

PROFESSOR BURNS.

The PRINCIPLES of MIDWIFERY.

By JOHN BURNS, C. M.

Regius Professor of Surgery, in the University of Glasgow, &c. &c.

The Fifth Edition. In 8vo. Price 14*s.* in Boards.

POPULAR DIRECTIONS for the TREATMENT of the DISEASES of WOMEN and CHILDREN. By JOHN BURNS, C. M.

In 8vo   Price 9*s.* in Boards.

MR. S. COOPER.

A DICTIONARY of PRACTICAL SURGERY; comprehending all the most interesting Improvements up to the present Period; also an Account of the Instruments, Remedies, and Applications employed in Surgery; the Etymology and Signification of the principal Terms; a copious Bibliotheca Chirurgica; and a Variety of original Facts and Observations. By SAMUEL COOPER. The Third Edition, revised, corrected, and enlarged. In one thick Volume 8vo. Price 1*l.* 4*s.* Boards.

The FIRST LINES of the PRACTICE of SURGERY, designed as an Introduction for Students, and a concise Book of Reference for Practitioners. By S. COOPER. 4th Edition, very much improved and enlarged, with several new Plates, in 2 Vols. 8vo. 1*l.* 10*s.* Bds.

DR. COOKE ON NERVOUS DISEASES.

In Two Vols. Volume I. Price 12*s.* bds.

ON APOPLEXY, including Apoplexia Hydrocephalica, or Water in the Head; with an Introductory Account of the Opinions of ancient and modern Physiologists, respecting the Nature and Uses of the Nervous System.

By JOHN COOKE, M.D. F.A.S.

The HISTORY and METHOD of CURE of the various Species of PALSY; being the first Part of the second Volume of a Treatise on Nervous Diseases.

By JOHN COOKE, M.D. F.A.S.

In 8vo. Price 6*s.* Boards.

MR. CARMICHAEL.

OBSERVATIONS on the Symptoms and Specific Distinctions of VENEREAL DISEASES; interspersed with Hints for the more effectual prosecution of the present Inquiry into the uses and abuses of Mercury in their Treatment. By RICHARD CARMICHAEL, M.R.I.A. In 8vo. Price 9*s.* boards.

An ESSAY on the VENEREAL DISEASES, which have been confounded with SYPHILIS, and the Symptoms which exclusively arise from that Poison. Illustrated by Drawings of the Cutaneous Eruptions of true Syphilis, and the resembling Diseases. By RICHARD CARMICHAEL, M. R. I. A. &c. In Quarto, with coloured Plates, Price 1*l.* 18*s.* Boards.

MR. A. COOPER AND MR. TRAVERS.

SURGICAL ESSAYS.

By ASTLEY COOPER, F.R.S. Surgeon to Guy's Hospital, and BENJAMIN TRAVERS, F.R.S. Surgeon to St. Thomas's Hospital.

Part I. the Third Edition, Price 10*s.* 6*d.* Boards. Part II. 2nd Edit. in 8vo. price 10*s.* 6*d.*

A SYNOPSIS of the DISEASES of the EYE, and their TREATMENT; to which are prefixed, a short ANATOMICAL DESCRIPTION, and a Sketch of the PHYSIOLOGY of that Organ.

By BENJAMIN TRAVERS, F.R.S. Surgeon to St. Thomas's Hospital.

In 1 Vol. 8vo. with six highly finished coloured Engravings, price 1*l.* 5*s.* boards.

An INQUIRY into the PROCESS of NATURE in repairing Injuries of the Intestines, illustrating the Treatment of penetrating Wounds and Strangulated Hernia.

By BENJAMIN TRAVERS, F. R. S.

1 vol. 8vo. with Engravings by Stewart. 15*s.* Bds.

DR. CLUTTERBUCK.

OBSERVATIONS on the NATURE and TREATMENT of the EPIDEMIC FEVER, at present prevailing in the Metropolis, as well as in most Parts of the United Kingdom. To which are added, Remarks on some of the Opinions of Dr. Bateman, in his late Treatise on this Subject.

By HENRY CLUTTERBUCK, M. D.

In 8vo. price 8*s.* Boards.

MR. CARLISLE.

An ESSAY on the DISORDERS of OLD AGE, and on the Means for prolonging Human Life. By ANTHONY CARLISLE, F. R. S. F. S. A. F. L. S. &c. &c. The Second Edition, with several important additions. In 8vo. Price 5*s.* Boards.

The HUNTERIAN ORATION, delivered before the Royal College of Surgeons, in London, on Monday, February 21, 1820. By ANTHONY CARLISLE, F.R.S. F.S.A. F.L.S. &c. In 4to. Price 5*s.* sewed.

DR. J. CLARKE.

COMMENTARIES on some of the most IMPORTANT DISEASES of CHILDREN. PART THE FIRST,—Containing Observations on the Mortality of Children—on Diet—Dentition—Convulsive Affections—Inflammation of the Brain—Hydrocephalus internus—and Epilepsy. By JOHN CLARKE, M. D. &c. In royal 8vo. price 10*s.* 6*d.* Boards.

DUBLIN MEDICAL TRANSACTIONS.

TRANSACTIONS of the ASSOCIA-TION of Fellows and Licentiates of the King's and Queen's College of Physicians in Ireland. Vol. I. price 14s., Vol. II. price 16s., and Vol. III. price 14s. Boards.

DR. FARRE.

A TREATISE on some PRACTICAL POINTS relating to the DISEASES of the EYE. By the late JOHN CUNNINGHAM SAUNDERS.

To which is added, a short Account of the Author's Life, and his Method of curing the Congenital Cataract, by his Friend and Colleague, J. R. FARRE, M. D.

Third Edition, with Additions, in Demy 8vo. with Engravings. Price 14s. plain, and 1l. 5s. with the Plates coloured.

The MORBID ANATOMY of the LIVER, being an Inquiry into the Anatomical Character, Symptoms, and Treatment of certain Diseases which Impair or Destroy the Structure of that Viscus. By J. R. FARRE, M. D.

Part I. and II. in Imperial Quarto, Price 15s. each. Part III. is preparing for the Press.

PATHOLOGICAL RESEARCHES in MEDICINE. By J. R. FARRE, M. D.

Essay I. On MALFORMATIONS of the HUMAN HEART; illustrated by numerous Cases, and Five Plates, in royal 8vo. Price 7s. Sewed.

Part II. is preparing for the Press.

DR. GOOCH.

A TREATISE on the HYDROCE-PHALUS ACUTUS, or Inflammatory Water in the Head. By LEOPOLD ANTHONY GOLIS, Physician and Director of the Institute for the Sick Children of the Poor at Vienna. Translated from the German, by ROBERT GOOCH, M.D.

MR. GOODWIN.

AN ACCOUNT of the various MODES of SHOEING HORSES, employed by different Nations; more particularly a Comparison between the English and French Methods. With Observations on the Diseases of the Feet, connected with Shoeing. By JOSEPH GOODWIN, Esq. Veterinary Surgeon to his Royal Highness the Prince Regent. In 8vo. with Plates, 12s. Bds.

MR. HARE.

A VIEW of the STRUCTURE, FUNCTIONS, and DISORDERS of the STOMACH, and ALIMENTARY ORGANS of the HUMAN BODY; with Physiological Observations and Remarks upon the Qualities and Effects of Food and fermented Liquors. By THOMAS HARE, F.L.S. &c. Fellow of the Royal College of Surgeons in London. In 8vo. Price 12s. Bds.

DR. HASLAM.

SOUND MIND, or Contributions to the Natural History and Physiology of the Human Intellect. By JOHN HASLAM, M. D. late of Pembroke Hall, Cambridge; formerly President of the Royal Medical, Natural History, and Chemical Societies of Edinburgh. 8vo. 7s. Bds.

MR. HOWSHIP.

PRACTICAL OBSERVATIONS on the Symptoms, Discrimination, and Treatment of some of the most common Diseases of the lower Intestines and Anus; to which are added, some Suggestions upon a new and successful Mode of correcting habitual Confinement in the Bowels, to ensure their regular Action without the Aid of Purgatives. By J. HOWSHIP, Member of the Royal College of Surgeons in London; Member of the Medico-Chirurgical Society; and Corresponding Member of the Société Médicale d'Emulation, in Paris. 2d Edit. 8vo. Price 8s. 6d. Bds.

PRACTICAL OBSERVATIONS in SURGERY and MORBID ANATOMY. With Cases, Dissections, and Engravings. By JOHN HOWSHIP. In 8vo. Price 18s. Bds.

DR. M. HALL.

CASES of a SERIOUS MORBID AF-FECTION, principally incident to Females after Delivery, Abortion, &c. and arising from Uterine Hæmorrhagy, undue Venæsection, Menorrhagia, protracted Lactation, Diarrhœa, Aphthæ, Constipation, Scybalæ, or other Causes of Exhaustion and Irritation.

By MARSHAL HALL, M.D. F.R.S.E. &c. price 4s.

By the same Author,

A DESCRIPTIVE, DIAGNOSTIC, and PRACTICAL ESSAY on DISORDERS of the DIGESTIVE ORGANS and GENERAL HEALTH; being an Attempt to prosecute the Views of Dr. Hamilton and Mr. Abernethy, and a Second Edition of the Essay on the Mimoses, with Additions. In 8vo. price 7s. boards.

On DIAGNOSIS, in Four Parts.—The Phœnomena of Health and Disease.—Of the Diseases of Adults. —Of Local Diseases.—Of the Diseases of Children, in 8vo. 16s. boards.

MR. HUTCHINSON.

CASES of TIC DOULOUREUX successfully treated. By BENJAMIN HUTCHINSON, Member of the Royal College of Surgeons of London, &c. Price 3s. 6d.

DR. MARCET.

AN ESSAY on the CHEMICAL HISTORY and MEDICAL TREATMENT of CALCULOUS DISORDERS.

By ALEXANDER MARCET, M.D. F.R.S. 2d Edit. Royal 8vo. with Plates. 18s. Boards.

DR. MAGENDIE.

PHYSIOLOGICAL and MEDICAL RESEARCHES into the Causes, Symptoms, and Treatment of Gravel. Translated from the French of F. MAGENDIE, M.D. Professor of Anatomy, Physiology, &c. &c. at Paris. 12mo. 3s. 6d. Bds.

MEDICAL TRANSACTIONS, published by the College of Physicians in London. Vol. 6, in 8vo. with coloured Plates, Price 12s. Bds.

Also may be had, Vols. 1 to 5, Price 2l. 8s. Bds.

M. P. ORFILA.

DIRECTIONS for the TREATMENT
of PERSONS who have TAKEN POISON, and those in a state of Suspended Animation; together with the Means of detecting Poisons and Adulteration in Wine: also, of distinguishing Real from Apparent Death. By M. P. ORFILA. Translated from the French, by R. H. BLACK, Surgeon. The 2nd edit. In 1 vol. 12mo. 5s. Bds.

DR. POWELL.

The PHARMACOPŒIA of the ROYAL
COLLEGE of PHYSICIANS of LONDON, 1809. Translated into English, with Notes, &c. by R. POWELL, M.D. Fellow of the College, Physician to St. Bartholomew's and the Magdalen Hospitals.

A New Edition, revised and corrected. In 8vo. Price 12s. Boards.

MR. A. T. THOMSON.

The LONDON DISPENSATORY;
containing—1. Pharmacy—2. The Botanical Description, Natural History, Chemical Analysis, and Medicinal Properties, of the Substances of the Materia Medica.—3. The Pharmaceutical Preparations and Compositions of the Pharmacopœias of the London, Edinburgh, and Dublin Colleges of Physicians. The whole forming a practical Synopsis of Materia Medica, Pharmacy, and Therapeutics: illustrated with many useful Tables and Copper-plates of Pharmaceutical Apparatus.

By ANTHONY TODD THOMSON, F. L. S. In One large Vol. 8vo. (revised and altered according to the last Edition of the London and Edinburgh Pharmacopœias). 15s. Bds. 2d Edit.

*** This edition contains the synonyma of the names of the articles, in the French, German, Italian, Spanish, and East Indian languages.

DR. J. THOMSON.

An ACCOUNT of the VARIOLOID
EPIDEMIC, which has lately prevailed at Edinburgh and other Parts of Scotland; with Observations on the Identity of Chicken Pox with modified Small Pox; in a Letter to Sir James M'Grigor, Director General of the Army Medical Department, &c. &c. By JOHN THOMSON, M.D. F.R.S.E. &c. &c. &c. In 8vo. Price 10s. 6d. Bds.

THE FOLLOWING WORKS ARE PREPARING FOR PUBLICATION.

SURGICAL OBSERVATIONS; being
a Quarterly Report of Cases in Surgery. By CHARLES BELL.

The First Volume is already published, in 4 Parts, illustrated with Plates, Price 1l. 4s. This Volume contains Reports—Of the Treatment of Cancer by Compression—Of Soft Cancer—Of Ulcerations of the Throat which cause Suffocation—Of Tumors which arise from the Gums—Of Abscess and Fistula connected with the Urethra—Of the Structure and Diseases of the Prostate Gland—Of the Pulmonary Diseases which attend Surgical Operations—Of sounding for the Stone, where it is sacculated—Of Counter Fissure—Of the Nitro-muriatic Bath in Cutaneous Diseases, which resemble Syphilis, &c.—Of wounded Arteries—Of Fractures.

Part VI. will be published shortly.   Price 6s.

MEDICO-CHIRURGICAL TRANS-
ACTIONS, published by the Medical and Chirurgical Society of London. Volume XI. Part II.—Vols. 1 to 10 may be had, Price 9l. 3s. Boards, illustrated with Plates.

Also, Volume XI. Part I.   Price 9s. Bds.

MR. C. M. CLARKE.

OBSERVATIONS on those DISEASES
of FEMALES, which are attended by DISCHARGES.

By CHARLES MANSFIELD CLARKE, Member of the Royal College of Surgeons; and Lecturer on Midwifery in London.

In royal 8vo. illustrated with Plates.

Part the Second, including the White Opake Discharge, the Watery Discharge, and Purulent Discharge. The Diseases comprehended under these heads are, Inflammation of the Cervix Uteri—Cauliflower Excrescence of the Os Uteri—the Oozing Tumour of the Labia—Hydatids of the Uterus—Ulcerated Carcinoma, or Cancer of the Uterus—Ulceration and Abscess of the Vagina, together with some Observations upon disordered Menstruation.

Recently published,

A New Edition of Part I. of the above Work—On Mucous Discharges. In royal 8vo. with Plates. Price 1l. 1s. Bds.

DR. GRANVILLE.

MEMOIRS on the PRESENT STATE
of SCIENCE and SCIENTIFIC INSTITUTIONS in FRANCE: containing a Descriptive and Historical Account of the Royal Garden of Plants; the Royal Institute; the Polytechnic School; the Faculty of Sciences; the College of France; and the Cabinet of Mineralogy; the Public Libraries; the Medical School; and the Hospitals. With Plans of the latter never before published, &c. &c.

Interspersed with ANECDOTES and BIOGRAPHICAL SKETCHES of all the EMINENT CHARACTERS who have appeared in France during and since the Revolution, in the various Departments of Science. Accompanied with Observations upon their Writings, Inventions, Discoveries, and Public Conduct.

By A. B. GRANVILLE, M.D. F.R.S. F.L.S. M.R.I. In Two Vols. 4to.   Illustrated by Numerous Plates and Tables.

OBSERVATIONS

ON

THE NATURE AND CURE OF

DROPSIES,

AND PARTICULARLY ON

THE PRESENCE OF THE COAGULABLE PART OF THE BLOOD IN DROPSICAL URINE;

To which is added,

AN APPENDIX,

CONTAINING

SEVERAL CASES OF ANGINA PECTORIS,

WITH DISSECTIONS, &c.

BY

JOHN BLACKALL, M.D.

PHYSICIAN TO THE DEVON AND EXETER HOSPITAL, AND TO THE LUNATIC ASYLUM, NEAR EXETER.

THE THIRD EDITION, CORRECTED AND IMPROVED.

LONDON:

PRINTED FOR LONGMAN, HURST, REES, ORME, AND BROWN, PATERNOSTER-ROW.

1818.

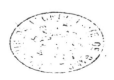

Printed by A. Strahan,
Printers-Street, London.

TO THE

PRESIDENT AND GOVERNORS

OF THE

DEVON AND EXETER HOSPITAL,

WHICH HAS FURNISHED

SOME OF THE MOST IMPORTANT OBSERVATIONS

CONTAINED IN THE FOLLOWING PAGES,

THIS WORK

IS VERY RESPECTFULLY INSCRIBED,

BY THEIR OBLIGED

AND OBEDIENT

HUMBLE SERVANT,

THE AUTHOR.

TABLE OF CONTENTS.

CHAPTER XV.

APPENDIX.

INTRODUCTION.

IT is my design in the following pages to treat of those accumulations of serous fluid which take place in the cellular membrane, and circumscribed cavities of the body, and are denominated dropsies. Their great variety renders some arrangement of them necessary for this purpose; whilst the obscurity of their own nature, and their complication with other disorders, throw many obstacles in the way of such an attempt.

There is one consideration, indeed, too obvious to be overlooked; namely, the seat of the accumulated fluid. Systematic writers have made great use of this distinction; and if a dropsy of the same cavity were always the same disease, there would be no need for any other. But a very slight attention to the subject is sufficient to disprove this supposition, and to show, not only that local dropsies originate in different injuries of the affected parts, but that even those extensive effusions which inundate at once almost every cavity of the body, do not always arise from the same constitutional cause.

Many of these are symptomatic of an unsoundness of the viscera, and in not a few instances seem to be connected with a mechanical obstruction to the circulating fluids. Others again are attributed with much probability to a watery state of the blood, and a feebleness of the exhalant and absorbent vessels ; whilst practical writers have noticed some cases of original dropsy entirely at variance with this doctrine, and in which the blood has been found remarkably inflamed.

The same conclusion may be derived from the extreme uncertainty and very inaccurate application of the remedies employed. Dr. Monro very candidly confesses this great defect. Dr. Cullen's words are still more remarkable.

Speaking of diuretics, he says : " It hap-
" pens unluckily, that none of these are of
" very certain operation ; neither is it well
" known, why they sometimes succeed, and
" why they so often fail ; nor why one me-
" dicine should prove of service, when an-
" other does not."

Such an inaccuracy in the direction of
remedies cannot well be imputed to any
thing but an obscurity in the disease ; and
that we confound, under the same title, different affections of the habit.

The older physicians did not lose sight
of this consideration ; and their writings
abound with distinctions founded on proximate causes, but particularly on the supposed state of the circulating fluids. Hence
the leucophlegmatia, the cachexy, the
scurvy of some authors, &c. which denote œdematous swellings differing from
each other, and from the common anasarca.
These terms have, indeed, on account of
the fanciful theories connected with them,
fallen into some neglect ; but nothing satisfactory has been substituted in their stead ;
and it must be acknowledged that we still
remain greatly in need of some rational dis-

tinctions of this kind, derived from the constitutional circumstances of the disease as well as its situation.

It has often occurred to me, that such an arrangement might be much facilitated, by a more accurate inquiry than has hitherto been made, into those remarkable properties of the urine, which characterize a large proportion of dropsies. Writers have spoken of the colour of that secretion, its quantity, its sediment; and it is a circumstance hardly credible that, amidst so much minute labour bestowed on these topics, the effect produced on it by the application of heat should have been so greatly overlooked. Yet the experiment is the easiest possible; and every practitioner may shortly convince himself beyond the possibility of doubt, that in a considerable number of dropsical cases the urine coagulates like diluted serum of the blood.

So extraordinary a phænomenon cannot be investigated with too much care; and the distinctions, which it seems capable of affording in nosology, are undoubtedly not to be neglected. But I wish, in the first place, to direct the attention of the reader to the fact itself, and to the notice which it has hitherto received.

———————

At St. Bartholomew's Hospital in 1795, there was admitted, under the care of my most respected preceptor, Dr. Latham, a patient, whom he mentions in his work on Diabetes, as affected with a remarkable and copious discharge of serum from the kidneys. *

In this person, at the time of his admission, I observed an emaciation of the whole body, with an œdema of the right leg only, a small and quick but not frequent pulse, an excessive feebleness and dejection of spirits, a sallowness of complexion, and a foul tongue. He complained, likewise, of a pain at the margin of the ribs on the left side, great thirst, loss of appetite, and occasional vomiting; and his bowels were much obstructed.

Two months before, he had been attacked by severe shiverings, and other febrile

* See Latham on Diabetes, p. 139.

symptoms, with vomiting and constipation, and had hardly quitted his bed till the period of his admission. The vomiting in particular had been troublesome, and at first almost incessant; and he had sometimes thrown up in that way small quantities of blood.

The urine was made in larger quantities than natural, and in the night more copiously than in the day time. Altogether it rather exceeded the solid and fluid ingesta, amounting to about seven pints in twenty-four hours.

A parcel of it was subjected to evaporation, with some expectation of obtaining a saccharine extract. To my great surprize, when the heat rose to 160° of Fahrenheit, the fluid became uniformly opaque and white, and a considerable precipitate took place, which, when strained, but not much dried, amounted in weight to more than half an ounce, from two quarts of urine, or about one ounce from the quantity discharged daily.

A similar effect was produced by nitrous acid.

The filtrated liquor on evaporation gave a very small extract, which did not contain any saccharine matter.

Dr. Latham, after exhibiting a few laxatives, which seemed to answer their purpose well, proceeded to the use of astringent medicines, and a blister to the loins, but without any good effect.

This patient quitted the Hospital, after remaining there about three months; and six weeks afterwards he died.

Facts of this nature have been but slightly alluded to by medical writers.

Dr. Fordyce asserts in his Elements, that if the kidneys be relaxed or stimulated, chyle, serum, coagulable lymph, and even the red part of the blood may be thrown out. This notice is so concise, that it is impossible to say what species of cases he had in his mind in the description.

Dr. Darwin, in the first volume of his Zoonomia, states, on the authority of Cotunnius, that there is a mucilaginous diabetes connected with the beginning of some dropsies. He adds, that it proves a temporary cure of the disorder. His words are as follows:

" There is a third species of diabetes, in
" which the urine is mucilaginous, and ap-
" pears ropy, in pouring it from one vessel
" into another; and will sometimes coagu-
" late over the fire. This disease appears
" by intervals, and ceases again, and seems
" to be occasioned by a previous dropsy in
" some part of the body. When such a col-
" lection is reabsorbed, it is not always
" returned into the circulation; but the
" same irritation that stimulates one lym-
" phatic branch to reabsorb the deposited
" fluid, inverts the urinary branch, and
" pours it into the bladder. Hence this
" mucilaginous diabetes is a cure, or the
" consequence of a cure, of a worse disease
" rather than a disease itself.

" Dr. Cotunnius gave half an ounce of
" cream of tartar, every morning, to a pa-
" tient who had the anasarca, and he voided
" a great quantity of urine, a part of which,
" put over the fire, coagulated, on the eva-
" poration of half of it, so as to look like
" the white of an egg. *De Ischiade Nervos.*

" This kind of diabetes frequently pre-

" cedes a dropsy, and has this remarkable
" circumstance attending it ; that it gene-
" rally happens in the night, as, during the
" recumbent state of the body, the fluid that
" was accumulated in the cellular mem-
" brane, or in the lungs, is more readily
" absorbed, as it is less impeded by its
" gravity.

" I have seen more than one instance of
" this disease. — Mr. D. a man in the de-
" cline of life, who had long accustomed
" himself to spirituous liquors, had swelled
" legs, and other symptoms of approaching
" anasarca : about once in a week or ten
" days, for several months, he was seized on
" going to bed with great general uneasi-
" ness, which his attendants resembled to
" an hysteric fit ; and which terminated in
" a great discharge of viscid urine ; his legs
" became less swelled, and he continued
" in better health for some days after-
" wards. I had not the opportunity to try
" if his urine would coagulate over the fire,
" when part of it was evaporated, which I
" imagine would be the criterion of this
" kind of diabetes ; as the mucilaginous
" fluid deposited in the cells and cysts of the

" body, which have no communication with
" the external air, seems to acquire, by
" stagnation, this property of coagulation by
" heat, which the secreted mucus of the in-
" testines and bladder do not appear to pos-
" sess, as I have found by experiment ; and
" if any one should suppose this coagulable
" urine was separated from the blood by the
" kidneys, he may recollect, that in the
" most inflammatory diseases, in which the
" blood is most replete, or most ready to
" part with the coagulable lymph, none of
" this appears in the urine." *

This great author would, without doubt,
have modified his opinion, had he made any
experiments himself, and would have ascertained that the coagulation, of which he
speaks, takes place long before the boiling
heat ; that it is not a temporary relief, but
a continued symptom of some dropsies, and
not merely at their beginning, but through
their whole course ; and that the curative
effort of nature is an urine not loaded with
serum, but almost devoid of it.

* Darwin's Zoonomia, vol. 1st, p. 316.

Vauquelin and Fourcroy, in two Memoirs on the Analysis of Human Urine, published in the Annales de Chimie *, have noticed the proportion of gelatinous matter and albumen, which often abound in that fluid, as capable of furnishing considerable evidence of the state of the constitution.

They inform us, that the urine, which is least gelatinous, is most coloured, has a stronger smell, and more urinary matter, and is in consequence less susceptible of fermentation or putridity; whilst that which is more gelatinous is likewise less coloured, and more disposed to the formation of ammonia, more speedily deposits flakes both by evaporation and spontaneous decomposition, and gives a cloud or precipitate. The former of these is a sign of good health, and the produce of complete digestion; the latter exists in weak subjects, and in cases where the digestive faculties are much injured.

They add, there is reason to believe, that these two states will one day furnish us with

* See Annales de Chimie, tom. 31. & 32.

facts of great utility in the healing art, and that a solution of tan will supply the means of distinguishing them.

These remarks, valuable as they are, do not, however, apply to any particular disorder ; and they refer more to the presence of an animal matter, detected by infusion of galls, than of albumen, as precipitated by less than the boiling heat. They come, however, from such high authorities, and are so nearly connected with my subject, that no apology can be necessary for inserting them in this place.

Mr. Cruickshank, in his appendix to Dr. Rollo's excellent work on Diabetes, notices the serous urine more precisely than any other author has done. *

He asserts, that it is a symptom of general dropsy, that sometimes this discharge differs but little from serum of the blood ; and that he has known a patient carried off by it in a few weeks.

Several writers on animal chemistry have since made the same distinction ; but there

---

* See Appendix to Rollo on Diabetes, p. 447. and 448.

is no author, as far as I am informed, who has discussed the subject in a practical manner *, or applied these observations to the treatment of the disease.

* The very able papers of Dr. Wells on this subject form an exception to the above remark; but as they did not appear till the first edition of this work was in the press, they could be noticed in an appendix only. It was thought most advisable to reprint that appendix in its original form; and to it I beg leave to refer the reader.

CHAPTER I.

IN the following remarks on dropsies, I intend to avail myself of the important distinctions suggested by Mr. Cruickshank.

That ingenious author asserts, that, in the general dropsy, the urine coagulates like diluted serum of the blood ; whilst in that which proceeds from unsound viscera, it is usually high-coloured and scanty, deposits on cooling a pink-coloured sediment, and does not coagulate either by heat or the nitrous acid.

This doctrine must be received with those limitations, which almost every opinion in medicine requires. The former of

these appearances is certainly often connected with visceral obstructions; the latter are sometimes, I believe, independent of
any such taint; and there are other states
of that secretion, in which it is neither
loaded with serum, nor scanty, high-coloured, and full of sediment, but occasionally, and in some particulars at least, runs
towards the contrary extreme.

These different conditions of the urinary
discharge seem to indicate a corresponding
difference in the constitutional affection, to
which they belong; and I entertain hopes,
that hereafter, and under a more accumulated experience, they may be found important guides in practice.

I shall consider them not exactly in the
order in which they have been here mentioned, but, for reasons which will soon
appear more evident, treat — First,

Of those dropsies, in which the urine is
not coagulable by heat.

Secondly, of those in which it is so coagulable, in a greater or less degree.

In looking at the former of these, our attention is naturally directed to the other
appearances of that secretion. It is in

some cases pale, crude, without sediment, even copious ; in some rather scanty, but otherwise differing little from the healthy state ; in many it is both high-coloured and scanty, grows extremely turbid on cooling, and deposits a copious sediment, more or less lateritious.

These differences of colour and sediment, varying as they do with diet, exercise, and the peculiarities of the individual, may be thought, perhaps, very imperfect, as the distinguishing characteristics of diseases ; I do not adduce them as such, but rather as a foundation for some practical remarks. Where diuretics are wanted, and a selection must be made, it seems but reasonable to look attentively to the actual state of the secretion. In dropsies it is rarely not concerned, and speaks forcibly of the internal state. Van Helmont, in his chapter, entitled *Ignotus Hydrops*, has even pronounced the seat of this disorder to be the kidneys themselves. I have therefore thought it right, in the present inquiry, not to neglect even these minute circumstances of the urinary discharge, although I acknowledge them to be of a value infinitely

c

less than the result furnished by the application of heat ; and my observations on them will be in some measure but a necessary introduction to this part of the subject.

For these purposes, I must request the attention of the reader to some cases related in detail, which I have thought to be the only proper mode of presenting to him facts hitherto so little noticed. He will thus be enabled to judge for himself.

CHAPTER II.

CASES OF DROPSY, IN WHICH THE URINE, NOT COAGULABLE BY HEAT, WAS PALE, CRUDE, AND WITHOUT SEDIMENT, SOMETIMES COPIOUS.——RE-MARKS.

CASE I.

M. T. ætat. 12, was just recovering from scarlatina, in which the inflammation of the skin had been severe, and the bowels unusually relaxed. She had quitted her bed a few days only, and on the evening preceding my visit, the ankles and knees had begun to swell.

There was a considerable degree of languor and loss of appetite, a quick and weak pulse, pain of the left side, a loose state of the bowels, and swelling of most of the joints, particularly the left knee, in the large bursa mucosa above which, there was a very evident fluctuation.

The urine was rather scanty, pale, and without sediment ; it was coagulable neither by heat nor nitrous acid, and in the slightest degree by the oxymuriate of mercury. Some precipitate was produced by the infusion of galls, and a copious flaky one by the acetate of lead.

True dropsical symptoms succeeded rapidly. In less than a fortnight she became universally anasarcous, and there was a fluctuation of water in the abdomen, with orthopnœa and frightful dreams. At length she spent several successive nights in her chair, unable to lie down. It was impossible to entertain any doubt of the presence of hydrothorax. During the whole of this time the urine, examined daily, gave no appearance of coagulum. When she was most opprest, it was remarkably diluted, and quite colourless.

The tincture of digitalis, continued to such an extent as to retard the pulse and occasion much pain across the forehead, afforded not the least relief. On the contrary, the symptoms seemed to be aggravated under its use. The bowels at length becoming very costive, she took some smart purges of jalap and scammony. All the bad symptoms were speedily removed by this plan, and she wholly recovered under the use of Peruvian bark.

CASE II.

Sarah Somerton, ætat. 45, Devon and Exeter Hospital, 1798.——Considerable anasarca, with a very feeble pulse, and loss of appetite ; urine pale, rather scanty, not coagulable by heat or nitrous acid, and depositing no sediment, but a slight cloud.

Six weeks before, she had been attacked by fever and a scarlet eruption, to which her dropsical symptoms had succeeded in a few days.

She derived immediate advantage from the bitter infusion and alkaline salt, as recommended by Sir John Pringle, and soon recovered.

CASE III.

M. S. ætat. 50.——Anasarca, ascites, cough, urine pale, rather copious, without sediment, and not at all coagulable by heat or nitrous acid.

These complaints had continued for some months, and she attributed them to cold.

She was benefited neither by squills, nor calomel, nor digitalis. I understood that she afterwards became jaundiced; but I am not informed of the event.

CASE IV.

J. T. ætat. 40, of a sallow countenance, laboured under cough, dyspnœa, pain in the region of the stomach, loss of appetite, and swellings of the legs.

He had been much exposed to changes of weather during the preceding winter, and lately had suffered from fever and several bleedings at the nose.

The sallowness of his complexion induced

me to order a few doses of calomel, which purged and debilitated him. His urine before and after this was uniformly pale, rather scanty, and without sediment. No coagulum was produced by heat or nitrous acid, and very little by the corrosive sublimate. The infusion of galls had some effect; and an unusually large precipitate took place on the addition of Goulard's Extract.

After some time he had a nightly orthopnoea, which made me suspect hydrothorax. His abdomen likewise enlarged.

Squills rendered him not the least service. Digitalis greatly debilitated him, and increased his symptoms; and once, soon after the use of this drug, his urine gave a slight and loose coagulum when it reached the boiling heat. Purging with elaterium and jalap seemed to relieve his breathing most. The legs discharged freely, and all the dropsical symptoms were thus removed, except the ascites, which continues, very little affected by any remedies. He is, however, regaining his strength and colour.

CASE V.

J. W. ætat. 70, of what is usually called a scorbutic habit, and rather asthmatical, was subject for two or three winters before his death to swelled legs, and a cough ; he was unable to lie down in bed, and waked up in distressing suffocations. During the summer these symptoms were much alleviated ; but in the winter 1805, the chest again became affected ; and there was very considerable anasarca of the lower extremities.

At that time I found his pulse eighty, quick, regular ; appetite good, alvine discharges natural, urine of a light colour, clear, without sediment, not at all coagulating by heat or nitrous acid, furnishing an unusually large precipitate on the addition of acetate of lead, and in quantity exceeding the healthy standard. He often made between one and two quarts in the night.

The tincture of squills was tried in this instance, without any good effect. The powder of digitalis was then given, by the advice of another practitioner. He took but two doses, of one grain each. His pulse immediately became irregular, which it had never been before, and his stomach very languid. About a week after, he died suddenly.

CASE VI.

J. N. ætat. 60, subject when young to psorophthalmia and scaly eruptions of the skin, and since that period to irregular attacks of gout, was likewise extremely fanciful and hypochondriacal, and had the misfortune of having all his complaints attributed to this last cause. Many of them appeared to me, however, to be much more deeply seated. These were, a pulse stronger in the right arm than in the left; dyspnœa and palpitations on motion, a tendency to deliquia on slight occasions; orthopnœa after the first sleep, with great agitation of mind and sense of suffocation returning several times through the night, and attended with such a faintness as induced his friends to be constantly urging him to the use of cordials, a permanent uneasiness in the region of the heart, which was increased by lying on the right side, and a short cough, with some irritation about the larynx, which did not, however, prevent him from taking a full inspiration. To these were added, severe complaints of the stomach, acidity, heartburn, oppression after food, irregular appetite, and an inclination for pastry and fruit, over which he had no kind of command. A bilious diarrhœa was frequently the consequence of such imprudence.

There was a very considerable degree of anasarca.

His urine was pale and copious, and often deposited red gravel immediately on being discharged. It did not in the least coagulate by heat or nitrous acid, nor did it furnish any saccharine extract. But it was once observed, that on keeping long, it gave out, instead of the putrid fœtor, rather a mouldy and acetous smell; which Vauquelin and Fourcroy assert to be as common a form of decomposition in urine as the putrescent.

It was obvious that the alkaline diuretics were the only ones likely to be of service.

But these he never could be brought to use to any extent, not even the soda water.

He consulted many physicians, and took squills, digitalis, mercury, without advantage; afterwards he gradually became more suffocated and dropsical, and died in that state, having been attacked, in consequence of indigestion, several weeks before his death, by a vertigo and fullness of the head, which terminated in a permanent weakness of the right arm.

CASE VII.

A. W. ætat. 58, had been subject for more than two years to frequent returns of pain in the right side, attended by cough and dyspnœa. These symptoms had latterly become fixed, with considerable anasarca, and a copious pale urine, not coagulable.

She derived not the least benefit from fox-glove, calomel, squills, or strong purges, and soon died.

The urine above described as pale, crude, and apparently diluted, is not very common in dropsical complaints.

No coagulation is produced by heat or nitrous acid. In two instances, however, where I made the experiment, the addition of the oxymuriate of mercury detected the presence of a small quantity of albumen.

In the same instances the infusion of galls caused a very partial coagulation, less, certainly, than is observed in many other dropsies; but what proportion it bears in extent to a similar effect in other disorders, and in some circumstances of apparent health, I am unable to say. It is a subject entitled to further enquiry.

The copious flaky precipitate, thrown down by the acetate of lead, consists of saline matter, and, probably in no small degree, of animal mucilage, of which it is a delicate test.

This state seems to be often connected with great and irretrievable injury of the internal organs; but by no means uniformly so: on the contrary, the first example of it here related is likewise one of the least complicated cases in the whole volume; and apparently originated in that mere feebleness, both of the surfaces concerned and of the constitution, to which all dropsies have been referred by some authors. I request the particular attention of the reader to it. The changes of the urine were carefully observed, because, at the time of its occurrence, I supposed that the watery accumulations following scarlatina were always accompanied by a serous state of that discharge. It will be of importance to bear in mind this evidence to the contrary; although I am by no means prepared to say, in what proportion similar examples occur.

The inefficacy of digitalis, in the same instance, is well worthy of notice, but will be discussed with greater propriety in a more advanced stage of the enquiry. It has not succeeded better in the other cases ; of course its use cannot be indifferent. Diuretics, indeed, generally speaking, promise more in a scanty and loaded urine, than in the diluted state of it here mentioned. The carbonate of potash, joined with a mild bitter, is the most likely to be successful.

Where the viscera are untainted, much is to be hoped for from brisk and stimulating purges, such as scammony and jalap, &c. but from which calomel is excluded, and a very speedy use of the most active tonics immediately after the evacuation of the water, or even before, and mixed with the evacuants.

The well-known electuary of Dovar is a formula of this kind, and probably owes its character in a great measure to the addition of the chalybeate. A general laxity and sallowness of complexion particularly call for this remedy.

It appears, also, that an habitually large quantity of pale urine, not relieving the disorder, but forming a part of it, is a very bad sign, since it precludes the use of many diuretics, is more especially hostile to digitalis, and indicates a completely broken state of health. Some authors have alluded to it under the name of diabetes insipidus.

The most probable correctives of this symptom are the alkalis and magnesia (for the urine has a great tendency to acescency in such a state); and at the same time the weakness of the whole habit requires a free use of fermented liquors, and a liberal diet.

The leucophlegmatia, connected with chlorosis, belongs more to this place than to any other. The urine is pale, and gives no coagulum; but it contains sometimes a white sediment.

There is no pretence for saying, that any viscus is in these instances unsound in its organisation; and they therefore form another example of œdematous swellings of the asthenic kind, in which the urinary discharge is not serous. And if the general health be improved by chalybeates, the œdema spontaneously disappears.

CHAPTER III.

CASES OF ASCITES AND HYDROCEPHALUS, IN WHICH
THE URINE WAS RATHER SCANTY, BUT IN OTHER
RESPECTS APPEARED TO DIFFER LITTLE, OR NOT
AT ALL, FROM THE HEALTHY STATE.—— DISSEC-
TION.——REMARKS.

THOSE accumulations which take place
in the smaller and less vital cavities, as, for
example, the hydrocele, do not probably for
a long period affect the urine; but sometimes even when the parts concerned are
more extensive or essential to life, still that
secretion does not appear to be materially
changed, except, perhaps, in quantity. Of
this the following cases of ascites and hydrocephalus are a sufficient proof.

CASE I.

Mary Ellet, ætat. 20, Devon and Exeter
Hospital, 1798. —— Ascites; anasarca of the

lower extremities, upper part of the body much emaciated; pulse soft and feeble; loss of appetite ; menstruation obstructed ; but, at the expected periods, a slight leucorrhæal discharge.

The urine was rather scanty, clear, of a natural colour, deposited a slight branny sediment, and did not at all coagulate either by heat or nitrous acid.

About six months before, a spontaneous diarrhœa had come on, attended by irregular wandering pains of the abdomen, and had been speedily followed by ascites. The anasarca made its appearance very soon after ; and during the whole of this period she had been obstructed.

Laxatives, as indeed might reasonably have been foreseen, occasioned great disturbance of the system with no relief. She benefited more by the tincture of squills, till an over-dose produced vomiting and diarrhœa, and she could never bear a repetition of that medicine. The bitter infusion with alkaline salt was then directed for her with great advantage; and under the use of Griffiths' Chalybeate Mixture she entirely recovered.

D

CASE II.

Mary Gibbons, ætat. 40, was admitted into the Hospital, 1799, on account of a confirmed syphilis, and whilst under an active mercurial course principally by friction, was seized with a violent diarrhœa attended by discharges of blood, to which succeeded an ascites and anasarca of the lower extremities with great weakness and loss of appetite.

The urine gave no coagulum by heat or nitrous acid. It was of a natural colour, rather scanty, and deposited an inconsiderable branny sediment.

By the use of the Peruvian bark with diuretic salt, it flowed in great quantity, the swellings were carried off, and she was enabled to return to her mercurial course with advantage.

CASE III.

N. G. ætat. 2, a poor scrophulous infant, was troubled with a purulent discharge from the meatus auditorius externus, to relieve which her mother gave her two grains of calomel for many successive nights; being the remainder of some powders that had been of service to another child. They purged her greatly, and at length affected her gums. The breath was observed to be very fœtid, and she slavered much, although no longer about her teeth. In a few days she became heavy, unwilling to sit up, and vomited at intervals.

About a week after, I visited her, and finding the pulse slow and intermittent, great pain in the head, a fixed pupil, convulsions, strabismus, and a general feebleness that forbad evacuations, I could entertain little or no hope.

Her urine, with difficulty preserved, was of a natural colour, clear, and deposited a slight branny sediment. It did not in the least coagulate by the application of heat or nitrous acid. Its quantity was considered to be rather diminished. She died two days after. The parents consented to the examination of the head.

We found the dura mater adhering rather firmly to the cranium, the veins of the pia mater unusually turgid, and that membrane itself rather inflamed ; the lateral ventricles of the brain distended with a clear fluid to the amount of more than three ounces, which became slightly clouded on the application of heat; the neighbouring parts very soft, and covered with red points ; and some water in the other ventricles, as well as in the basis of the skull.   The purulent discharge before mentioned arose from the meatus externus only, and no injury extended to the internal parts of the organ of hearing, or to the bones connected with it.

———————

These two cases of ascites followed a diarrhœa; and the accumulations in the abdomen were probably the immediate effect of that loss of tone in its membranes which such a discharge seems calculated to produce.   It is observable, likewise, that the anasarca was of the lower extremities only.

The principal indication here was of course to improve the strength ; and any attempts to carry off the accumulations would have been advisable, only as they coincided with this.

The second of these cases, as well as that of hydrocephalus, are examples of the bad effects of mercury; and, I believe, the event and appearances recorded in the latter are a much more common result of large doses of calomel, in infantile complaints and scrophulous habits, than is generally suspected.

The extreme youth of the patients, and the discharge being often involuntary, make it difficult to ascertain the qualities of the urine in hydrocephalus. On these accounts I am uncertain, whether even its quantity is usually much lessened.

Mercurial purges are known to relieve the early symptoms of that disease, originating probably in foulness of the bowels; but in the present instance such a plan would obviously have been misapplied. Is it possible to think that any other would have succeeded? The debility so often produced in children by the rash and indiscrimate employment of purges and mercurials, and which in them is so apt to fall upon the brain, renders this question not an unimportant one.

D 3

CHAPTER IV.

OF DROPSY, IN WHICH THE URINE, NOT COAGU-
LABLE BY HEAT, IS SCANTY, AND HIGH-COLOUR-
ED, BECOMES EXTREMELY TURBID ON COOLING,
AND DEPOSITS A COPIOUS SEDIMENT, MORE OR
LESS LATERITIOUS.

THE dropsy, considered to be indicative of diseased viscera, is characterized by an urine scanty and high-coloured, loaded with a red sediment, and depositing nothing on the application of heat.

It includes a great variety of instances of ascites, hydrothorax, and hydrops pericardii, united with anasarca, some examples of which are here subjoined.

SECTION I. — *Cases with Dissections.*

CASE I.

A. S. ætat. 40, ascites, very slight ana-sarca, jaundice, pain of the right side, cough, frequent return of bilious vomiting and diarrhœa ; urine scanty, high-coloured, containing a red sediment, not at all coagulating on the application even of boiling heat.

She had been attacked with inflammatory symptoms some weeks before, to which the dropsy had gradually succeeded.

Calomel and opium at night, with tincture of squill two or three times daily, soon relieved her complaints.

Even after this relief, however, chalybeates could not be borne ; but she derived advantage from the bitter alkaline infusion.

CASE II.

M. C. ætat. 15, ascites, anasarca, pain of the right side, fæces scarcely tinged with bile, urine high-coloured, scanty, foul, depositing a branny and lateritious sediment, not at all coagulable by heat.

I found that jalap and crystals of tartar rendered no service; but some mercurial ointment rubbed on the abdomen, and the vinegar of squill in proper doses, rapidly carried off the swellings.

She then took a chalybeate electuary and was entirely cured.

CASE III.

H. B. a woman of very intemperate habits, lay oppressed with an ascites, swellings of the legs, and some sense of suffocation. The urine was very dark-coloured, foul, lateritious, and not at all coagulable by heat. What placed her in more immediate danger, was a violent bilious vomiting, with constipation.

Calomel removed this obstruction, the swellings remained, but were soon after carried off by the use of tincture of squill, and she completely recovered.

CASE IV.

R. B. ætat. 60, very robust and bulky, who had never entirely recovered from the effects of the influenza 1803, began about two years since more decidedly to emaciate and lose strength; and when he consulted me again about ten months ago, he was labouring under the most extensive ascites I ever witnessed; and his body was reduced to a mere skeleton. He informed me that he had lost more than 100 lbs. weight in six months. He was completely jaundiced; his urine very turbid, loaded with the pink-coloured sediment and with bile, but not at all altered by heat; his bowels irritable; and he suffered much from pain in the right side.

There could be no doubt that his complaint originated in a scirrhus of the liver; and as little expectation that any benefit could be derived from medicine. However, the bringing on a slight salivation, which we found very difficult, certainly lessened the abdomen several inches; but that process debilitated him, and he could not persist in it. He was afterwards tapped several times, and died quite exhausted.

CASE V.

W. R. ætat. 40, returned from Holland, 1799, labouring under a quotidian ague. This was afterwards stopped by Peruvian bark; but dropsical swellings of the legs still remained, with ascites, pain and stitches at the margin of the ribs on the left side, frequent cough, shortness of breathing, urine very scanty, foul, high-coloured, and loaded with a branny and lateritious sediment. On being exposed to heat it gave no coagulum.

Some blue ointment rubbed on the abdomen, one grain of calomel every night, and suitable doses of vinegar of squill, completely carried off these symptoms, after slightly affecting the gums.

CASE VI.

An officer in the army, who had served at the battle of Vimeira, returned to this country not long after, suffering from a tertian ague and considerable anasarca, with fulness in the region of the spleen.

The urine was scanty, high-coloured, and contained much lateritious sediment. It gave no coagulum on the application of heat.

The ague, which had been in vain treated with bark, disappeared when the gums were made sore by mercurial friction; and the swellings were soon removed by the use of the bitter alkaline infusion.

CASE VII.

J. R. returned from Walcheren with an irregular ague, to stop which vain attempts had been made by large doses of cinchona, as well as the mineral solution.

He had a cough, pain of the left side,

enlargement of the spleen felt externally, lower extremities very œdematus, urine high-coloured, depositing much lateritious sediment, not coagulating by heat.

Calomel and mercurial ointment, continued till his gums were sore, greatly debilitated him, without suspending the paroxysm; and I found with regret that the urine under their use began to coagulate by heat.

Of the further progress of this case I am not informed, as he was removed to quarters at some distance; but I understand that he at length recovered.

CASE VIII.

In the effects of mercury on the system, this case is analogous to the preceding.

R. S. ætat. 50, sallow, emaciated, affected with pain of the right side, soreness and fulness of the epigastric region, cough, sanious sputa, swelled legs; urine high-coloured, very turbid, lateritious, and not giving the least coagulum.

Both digitalis and squills were tried

without much good effect. By mild mercurials he seemed at first benefited; but after the continued use of this mineral, and a soreness of the gums partly produced by friction, he immediately became bloated, and affected with marked signs of internal as well as diffused dropsy. The urine now again examined gave a coagulum under the boiling heat; and I cannot help fearing that mercury had some share in thus changing the type of the disease.

CASE IX.

Anne Molony, Devon and Exeter Hospital 1797, ætat. 40, anasarca; ascites, joined with much distention of the abdomen from flatulency; pain at the margin of the ribs on the right side; tongue rather foul; bowels costive; pulse regular; urine scanty, foul, containing a copious branny sediment, with some lateritious, not coagulable by heat.

She was likewise much troubled with varicose veins of the legs, from which a peculiar kind of uneasiness and vapour were often propagated as high as the stomach.

She had suffered from dropsical symptoms for nearly twelve months; and the ascites had been much more considerable than it was at the time of her admission. The tincture of squill in the dose of fifty drops, with one grain of calomel every night, gave relief very speedily; she likewise derived great benefit from bandages on the legs, and was soon discharged from the hospital, cured.

CASE X.

A. D. ætat. 48, who, like the subject of the preceding case, was much distressed by varicose veins, and a peculiar uneasiness propagated from them to the stomach, was attacked in the winter of 1798 with increased tumour and erysipelas of the legs, anasarca, cough, shortness of breathing, inability of lying on the left side, which was likewise painful, urine scanty, foul, depositing a branny and some lateritious sediment, not coagulable.

These symptoms had continued two months before I was consulted. She was entirely relieved by the same plan as had been successful in the preceding instance, with the addition of a blister to the side.

CASE XI.

G. R. ætat. 40, formerly a very stout and healthy man, had been affected, eight months before I was called to him, with obscure symptoms, of which an overflow of bile and pain of the right side were considered the most predominant. To these gradually succeeded emaciation, anasarca, irregular and intermittent pulse, palpitations, cough, copious expectoration of frothy bloody sputa, great dyspnœa, such complete orthopnœa as obliged him to pass whole nights in his chair, dreadful suffocations and deliquia after his first sleep, considerable difficulty of deglutition, a croopy sound in breathing much aggravated by the least exertion, a very anxious countenance and great agitation of mind, at length spasms of the muscles of the face,

and a near approach to the risus sardo-
nicus.   I need not add, that death soon
followed.

Through the whole of his disorder there
was a costive body, and a sense of fulness at the pit of the stomach, partially
relieved by strong purging.

His urine was very scanty, and contained a branny and pink-coloured sediment,
but did not in the least coagulate by heat.

The dissection, which we were permitted
to make, showed how much the causes of
this malady were beyond the reach of any
human skill, or even of reasonable conjecture.

On opening the body we found considerable adhesions of the lungs to the pleura
on the right side, some of them elongated,
others firm and close; no water on either
side of the chest; in the cavity of the pericardium about two ounces of fluid, coagulating on the application of heat almost
as strongly as the serum of the blood; that
portion of the membrane which was re-
flected over the heart, dull, thickened, and
marked with several spots of lymph.

The lungs were apparently sound when

examined externally, but on removing them we discovered behind the trachea, at its bifurcation, a scirrhous mass of the size of a large man's fist. It extended from that spot a considerable way into the substance of the right lung, principally surrounding the bronchial tube.

In two or three parts of it were more defined round soft masses, resembling lymphatic glands beginning to suppurate.

The lower part of the trachea, but particularly the right branch, was inflamed and covered internally with a thin red lymph. But there was no appearance of any ulceration of the inner membrane.

The larynx and upper part of the trachea natural.

In the abdomen we found a few adhesions of the liver to the diaphragm on the right side; and on the surface of that gland two or three small thickened spots, hardly amounting to a diseased structure; every other part natural.

E

CASE XII.

H. L. ætat. 60, ascites; anasarca; cough with frothy crude expectoration, and pain of the left side; some difficulty of lying down in bed; pulse nearly natural; urine high-coloured, scanty, very foul, with a lateritious sediment, and not coagulable by heat. These symptoms had been forming for six months.

The tincture of squill carried off all appearance of dropsy; but some cough and pain of the side still remained.

CASE XIII.

S. B. ætat. 60, pain of the left side, reaching from the axilla to the hip; cough, with expectoration of a ropy mucus; some orthopnœa; difficulty of lying on the right side; palpitations; disturbed sleep; hurried dreams; purple lips; loaded and distressed countenance; pulse 80, regular; urine very scanty, depositing a branny and lateritious sediment, not coagulable.

Notwithstanding the absence of ana-sarca, there seems to be no reason to doubt that this was a case of hydrothorax.

A blister was applied, and the vinegar of squill given every eight hours.

The urine shortly became clear ; and all her complaints on the chest disappeared.

CASE XIV.

J. Penny, ætat. 62, Devon and Exeter Hospital, 1800. Great and univeral ana-sarca; dyspnœa; cough; orthopnœa; suffo-cations after the first sleep ; pain of the left side, and difficulty of lying on it ; urine scanty, high-coloured, foul, with a lateritious sediment, but not coagulable.

A blister, and four grains of the powder of squill, repeated at the interval of six hours, completely removed his symptoms, and he was discharged cured.

CASE XV.

L. C. ætat. 60, greatly debilitated in her nerves, and of a sallow complexion, after

E 2

having suffered from several attacks that were called bastard peripneumony, fell into a state of chronic cough and dyspnœa, great difficulty of walking up stairs, and fits of orthopnœa, with a tendency to deliquium about three o'clock in the morning.

There was no œdema of any part of the body ; pulse 90, regular ; urine not high-coloured, but scanty, depositing a white sediment, with some lateritious, and not coagulating by heat.

Twenty-five drops of the vinegar of squill, three times daily, rendered service, but very imperfectly, till one grain of calomel was added every night. The urine then flowed, and the dyspnœa entirely disappeared.

She has since been obliged occasionally to have recourse to the same medicines, and has certainly gained much ground.

More than two years have now elapsed since I first prescribed for her.

CASE XVI.

E. N. ætat. 48, when she consulted me, laboured under the following symptoms ; a weak and intermittent pulse ; palpitations ; face bloated and purple, with much anxiety of countenance, dyspnœa, orthopnœa, hurried dreams ; legs very œdematous and painful ; urine scanty, foul, loaded with a pink-coloured sediment, not coagulating.

These symptoms could not be mistaken ; they were carried off very rapidly by tincture of squills, with the addition of one grain of calomel at night.

She quitted my neighbourhood soon, and died about twelve months afterwards.

CASE XVII.

J. L. who had been thought in the spring of 1807 to labour under an inflammation both of the lungs and liver, and had been properly treated in consequence on a strictly

E 3

antiphlogistic plan, had remaining abuot him, during the summer, some cough, dyspnœa, and stricture on the chest. In the autumn a swelling of the legs came on, and such severe symptoms, as could leave no doubt of the existence of hydrothorax ; great dyspnœa, a total inability of lying down in bed, and after his first sleep even in his chair, the most horrible spasms, pulse 100, weak, but regular, urine scanty, high-coloured, foul, loaded with a pink-coloured sediment, not coagulating by heat.

He had tried digitalis with bad effect. I ventured in this urgent state to encourage the hope of relief by the tincture of squill, accompanied by a mild mercurial course. He bore the increase of the dose to sixty drops ; and then, at the moment at which his gums became sore, a copious diuresis took place. He was soon able to lie horizontally in bed, and to walk up and down stairs.

Between a fortnight and three weeks after the discontinuance of medicine, he complained one night of some little dyspnœa, and the next day, whilst walking across the room, dropt down and expired instantly.

CASE XVIII.

J. E. of a remarkably stout and robust chest and very active, ætat. 55, was affected, when I was called to him in January 1803, with the following symptoms; an irregular and intermittent pulse, a fluttering at the pit of the stomach, a harsh cough and mucous expectoration, great dyspnœa on motion, orthopnœa increasing after the first sleep to an agony both of body and mind which I never saw equalled in any other instance, extremities greatly swelled, purple and loaded countenance, the urine scanty, high-coloured, depositing a branny and pink-coloured sediment, not coagulable by heat.

About nine months before, he had been attacked by the influenza at that time epidemic, and then had suffered severely from pain of the right side and cough.

Through the summer, this last symptom had continued with dyspnœa, and a little tendency to dropsy, all which increased in the beginning of the winter, previously to my being consulted.

The tincture of squill, in the dose of thirty-five drops, repeated every eight hours, acted so speedily, that in a few days his urine became pale, limpid, and copious. The œdema was carried off, and the breathing quite relieved. The pulse likewise became more regular.

Through the ensuing summer he went on well; but the next winter his symptoms several times returned, and were as often checked by the same remedy.

When they were once more obstinate than usual, a little calomel was added, and the salivary glands and the kidneys became affected at the same time.

The digitalis was tried without any good effect.

At length after a period of more than two years, whilst apparently free from any dropsical symptoms, he died suddenly.

He had spent the early part of his life in the East Indies, where he had suffered much from the complaints peculiar to that climate. Since his return to England, however, he had become very strong, and capable of great exertions in field sports. It is, therefore, less material to add, that more than twenty years before, he had received a wound by a musquet shot in the thorax, near the left shoulder. He immediately expectorated large quantities of blood, became emphysematous, and for many months was thought consumptive. After a lapse of several years, the ball showed itself under the skin of the loins, and there continued during life.

CASE XIX.

L. G. ætat. 70, of a gouty habit, had laboured for several months under the following obscure symptoms ; a sense of bloating and fluttering at the pit of the stomach, with costive bowels, dyspnœa and faintness on motion, particularly on going up stairs, yet rather lessened than aggravated after dinner, not the least degree of orthopnœa or nightly suffocation, pulse from 120 to 130 in the minute, irregular and intermittent, which state of the circulation

had continued ever since he had been attacked by the influenza three years before.
There was very slight œdema of the legs.

The urine was likewise worthy of notice,
which, although not considered to be scanty,
was made frequently, in small quantities at
a time, and was very turbid and excessively
overloaded with a lateritious sediment.   It
did not coagulate on the application of
heat.

All these circumstances, notwithstanding
the quantity of the urine, convinced me,
that an internal dropsy existed.   The effect
of the remedy prescribed was a still more
convincing proof of this ; for, in consequence of the exhibition of squills, much
pale urine was voided, and immediate relief
obtained.

The same advantage was several times
afterwards derived from it, the moment the
water became much loaded.

Two winters since, in addition to his other
complaints, he had loss of appetite, nausea
aggravated by the medicine, bilious tinge
of the skin and eyes, and a feeling very distressing to himself of fluctuation of water
at the lower part of the sternum.   Small

doses of digitalis somewhat relieved him; but he relapsed, and soon after bore squills, united with opium, and was greatly benefited.

The horizontal posture preferred by this patient, and the sense of fluctuation perceived by himself, always convinced me that he laboured under a hydrops pericardii.

The complaints on his chest have now for more than two years entirely left him, having been succeeded by gout in the extremities, and a severe fit of the gravel.

CASE XX.

R. L. ætat. 60, sallow, but not jaundiced, had suffered for many months from gradually increasing dropsical symptoms, with a cough, ropy expectoration, great dyspnœa, some orthopnœa, and suffocations after the first sleep, pulse regular, the alvine discharges often nearly devoid of bile, urine scanty, foul, with a lateritious sediment, not coagulating by heat. He had tried in London a variety of remedies under very able practitioners, without the least good effect, particularly digitalis and strong purges.

I directed for him the vinegar of squills; and he had not taken it above a fortnight, before he was completely relieved both from his anasarca and the affection of his breath.

His own irregular habits and cold several times brought him into the same state again, and he was as often restored by the same means. A little calomel likewise rendered him service; but he could not be persuaded to go through a course of it.

Tonics, either bark or steel, had a tendency in every stage of his complaint to aggravate the symptoms.

After three years he died with jaundice and decided marks of a diseased liver.

CASE XXI.

Elizabeth Drawer, ætat. 60, Devon and Exeter Hospital, March, 1810. Universal anasarca; legs affected with a considerable erysipelas and deep sloughing sores; ulcers

on the sacrum and hips; pulse 110, weak,
irregular, intermittent; dyspnœa; nightly
suffocations; loose bowels; urine brown,
scanty, foul, containing a branny sediment,
with some lateritious. It did not in the
least coagulate by heat.

These symptoms had been forming two
months, and she attributed them to cold.
The tincture of squill increased the quantity
of urine, rendering it likewise pale and
perfectly without sediment. The legs were
consequently somewhat reduced, and the
breath very materially relieved; but the
ulcerations, aggravated by her unwieldy
habit, spread to a great extent, and soon
put a period to her life.

On examining the body the next day, we
found a small quantity of turbid fluid in the
abdomen; the liver much harder and somewhat smaller than natural, and the lower
edge slightly curled and bent forwards. Its
substance, when divided, exhibited no very
peculiar structure, but an unusual degree
of firmness and solidity. This Dr. Baillie
considers the first step towards the tuberculated liver, more commonly called scir-

rhous; the other viscera of the abdomen sound.

In the thorax, the lungs were sound, but adhering in several places to the pleura; about a pint and a half of pale fluid in each of its cavities, and somewhat more than the natural quantity in the pericardium.

The fluid taken from the cellular membrane by incision was a very diluted serum, hardly changing colour on being raised to boiling heat, and on evaporation throwing off a few films. The thoracic and pericardial fluids were less diluted, becoming opaque at about 160°.

The changes discovered on dissection, in this instance, are certainly neither far advanced nor unusual; but they are, perhaps, on those very accounts the more instructive, and point out to us in what an early stage of a scirrhus of the liver, hydrothorax, as well as anasarca, may take place.

SECTION II.

General Remarks on the preceding Cases, and particularly on the Dropsy that attends the intermittent and Walcheren Fevers.

FROM the preceding statement it is evident, that in a considerable proportion of dropsies, the urine, although apparently loaded with animal matter, does not contain albumen in such a form as to be detected by the test of heat. It will be found, even before much anasarca occurs, scanty, very high-coloured, made frequently and in small quantities. It grows extremely turbid on cooling, and deposits a copious sediment, which is lateritious and branny in various proportions, the former usually predominating and largely crystallized. A sediment of this sort terminates the paroxysms of intermittents and of gout, but is here rather symptomatic than critical, although it often appears in larger quantity, and of a brighter pink-colour than is customary in either.

To prevent the necessity of repetition, I have reserved it to this place to state, that on frequent trials a large extract has remained after evaporation, and a copious precipitate been thrown down by the infusion of galls, but none by nitrous acid. The oxymuriate of mercury likewise has sometimes produced a coagulum much resembling the effect of heat in some slighter cases of dropsy, where the urine is coagulable by that test. It appeared to me to be, in a great measure at least, albumen, as I have likewise stated it to be in the cases alluded to, page 28. If so, the precipitate caused by infusion of galls is not wholly gelatinous. *

This urine, when recent, reddens vegetable blues, but speedily putrefies. By a few experiments made with the other common re-agents, pure ammonia, the muriate of barytes, and acetate of lead, it likewise appears to contain rather a large propor-

* See Dr. Bostock on the Analysis of Animal Fluids, *Edinburgh Medical and Surgical Journal*, vol. 1st, p. 238, &c., and the same author on the Gelatine of the Blood, *Medico-Chirurgical Transactions*, vol. 1st, p. 72, &c.

tion of the saline matters which usually enter into the composition of this secretion, as indeed might be expected from its scantiness and want of dilution. The precipitate caused by the last was sometimes very large, and I suppose in these, as in many other instances, is greatly increased by the mucilage of the urine. *

It may be proper to add, that when the urine clears, and recovery is taking place, it is equally devoid of coagulum, probably with much less tendency to it than during the violence of the disease.

The reader has, I trust, gone before me in observing, that the examples above selected furnish a considerable variety, not only in the extent and seat of the watery accumulations, but also in the severity of the visceral obstruction and in the possibility of cure.

I do not see amongst them one instance of anasarca, unconnected with some injury of the breast or abdomen or some dropsy of those parts ; and I believe that such an anasarca rarely, if ever, does assume the

* See the work last quoted, p. 73 and 74.

F

form described in this chapter. The same assertion may be made of the hydrocephalus, and particularly of that sudden metastasis to the brain, which often occurs in original dropsies.

In cases I. II. III. IV. the principal symptom is an ascites, which with great appearance of justice is to be attributed to obstructions of the abdomen, particularly the liver, and which gentle courses of mercury with diuretics, as squills or the carbonate of potash joined with some bitter infusion, not uncommonly relieve. The carbonate is to be preferred to the subcarbonate, as being more palatable, but I am not aware that its diuretic effects are superior.

The three following, V. VI. VII., are examples of dropsy attending intermittent fever; and in two of them there was an evident enlargement of the left hypochondrium, in which the spleen seems to have been principally concerned; more, probably, by an accumulation of blood in its substance, than by a scirrhus, or in the first stages any active inflammation.

When such a case occurs, it is not al-

13

ways easy to say to what extent the mischief may have spread, and whether the texture of the affected parts has been much injured. The prognostic must of course be doubtful. If no entire disorganization has taken place, great benefit is sometimes derived from a course of mercury cautiously conducted. The bitter alkaline infusion is likewise a very excellent remedy; and under this plan I have seen the visceral obstruction and watery swellings, and even the ague, disappear at the same time.

In the more aggravated circumstances of this disorder, particularly after the Walcheren remittent, mercury often fails; and if given in any other way than as a purge, has been thought injurious. Its bad effects partly, perhaps, depend on a greater tendency to suppuration in such cases, from which even the lungs are not excluded, as I have more than once witnessed on dissection. But it seems likewise probable that the dropsy which supervenes on the Walcheren fever, especially after the dysentery and in exhausted subjects, is itself differently modified from that which attends the common ague; in short, that there com-

F 2

bines itself with the disease a truly hydropic diathesis, as shown by the quantity of albumen in the urine, a state of health this which mercurial courses often aggravate and even produce.

An altered texture of the blood, the consequence of the Walcheren remittent and of calomel exhibited for its cure, has been mentioned by Dr. Wright in his work on that complaint, and considered by him to be the cause of many of those dropsies which ensued.   He has even on this principle founded an arrangement of them, to which I refer the reader, as being not wholly dissimilar to mine, although he has not availed himself of the same signs. *

The phenomena occurring in case VII. first led me to suspect the danger of converting the common symptomatic swellings to a worse type by the too liberal use of mercury.   That which immediately follows, namely, VIII., adds great probability to this opinion ; and I believe it will be found to be fully proved in the succeeding pages of this volume.

* See Wright on the Walcheren Remittent, p.149 to179.

SECTION III.

On the Hydrothorax, its symptoms, causes, and cure by squills, calomel, &c.

IN the last nine of the remaining cases, namely, from XII. to XXI., the most marked and distressing circumstance of the disorder was the pressure of water in the thorax or pericardium, united very commonly with an anasarca extensively diffused, and still more with unsoundness of the viscera; but the favourable termination of case XIX. proves that it is not always so united. The utmost extent of a lateritious sediment was in this instance dependent on an effusion, in which the membranes appear to have been the parts affected, the glands probably being sound.

Generally, a loaded high-coloured urine is amongst the first symptoms. A slight œdema soon begins to show itself, with a harsh cough, attended by ropy expectoration, dyspnœa particularly increased on moving up stairs, and often such a sense of stricture or pain on one side of the chest, as rather encourages the opinion of some inflammatory action; and this appears to me more particularly probable, when I recollect that several elderly persons, whom I visited, fell into the hydrothorax after the influenza of 1803; and the first attacks are usually in the winter season. More decided signs of obstruction to the circulation at length show themselves; a purple, loaded, very anxious countenance, an irregular pulse, palpitations of the heart, a fluttering at the pit of the stomach, nightly orthopnœa with hurried dreams and all its aggravated sufferings.

Costiveness and flatulency are observed to a considerable degree, and not so much a loss of appetite as an oppression after food. The fæces are in many instances but partially tinged with bile; and frequently a true ascites is added to the other accumulations. Sallowness is not an unusual sign, and occasionally some degree of jaundice; but it is to be noticed that the patient is not commonly cachectic, or of a bloated pale complexion, to which appearance the *faciei pallor* of Dr. Cullen, that forms part of his definition of hydrothorax, seems particularly to allude.* If he directs himself properly, abstains from intemperate diet, and has a medical attendant, who will not force an unsound system by bark and chalybeates, he usually passes the ensuing summer in a tolerable state of health, and is disposed to flatter himself with the idea of a complete recovery. But he is shortly undeceived. The next return of cold weather, or the slightest irregularities even in the mean time, bring back all his complaints, but particularly that loaded state of the urine, which I have known to give the first warning of a relapse. At length medicine begins to lose its effect. After the termination of each attack, he is found to be more and more emaciated, and in a few years dies either suddenly or oppressed by an increasing suffocation, and probably during the prevalence of an east wind. Every such patient soon learns by experience to consider that as his greatest enemy. Rarely

* Cullen's Synopsis, vol. 2d, p. 278.

F 4

after being repeatedly relieved he seems to overcome his complaint.

The series of symptoms, above detailed, must be allowed to carry with it a strong presumption of visceral disease. Undoubtedly many of the appearances can only be explained on the supposition of a fluid collected in some cavity of the chest, or the cellular membrane of the lungs; and the sudden relief of the breathing by diuretics strongly confirms this opinion. But the increasing emaciation, the sallowness, the pulse never made uniform, the visceral countenance, &c. instruct us to consider these extravasations generally as mere symptoms, although prominent ones, and the cause to be more deeply rooted in great glandular unsoundness. The liver is more frequently accused than any other gland. Its size, its importance in the animal economy, the effect which a free mode of living is well known to have on it, the partial secretion of bile, and other symptoms unnecessary to be repeated, seem to prove that this accusation is often just. It is likewise rendered probable by several of these cases, particularly XX. and XXI., that some hepatic obstructions produce, even in their early stages, a disposition to hydrothorax, which is very much under the influence of medicine, till the original malady completely exhausts the patient. Such accumulations are naturally to be expected by us, when we recollect the situation of the unsound part so near to the lungs, the immediate connection which it has with the large blood vessels, the sympathy in short which is well known to subsist even in common inflammations between the organs above and those below the diaphragm. The bulk likewise and hardness of so large a scirrhus, acting almost like an extraneous body or dead weight attached to that muscle, will give great impediment to its movements; and all the bad consequences of an obstructed respiration and circulation through the lungs must necessarily ensue. Amongst these, a tendency to inflammation in full habits is frequently not the least; and the vessels will partially attempt to unload themselves by an increased exhalation.

I have observed, however, in such cases, (and the dissection in case XXI. particularly confirms this observation,) that the hydrothorax sometimes comes on earlier, and is more severe than the ascites. It does not so readily appear why this should ever take place ; all arguments drawn from the situation and structure of the parts would lead us to expect the contrary ; nor would the fact itself be of much practical importance, except as the presence of water in the chest, under certain circumstances, may lead to a suspicion of scirrhus of the liver, before it is unequivocally detected by its peculiar signs.

The pink-coloured sediment, so often mentioned, is considered by Mr. Cruickshank in some measure to characterize a scirrhous liver. Beyond any doubt it does not so universally. In case XI. this sediment was present ; and yet the injury was found to be seated in the lymphatics at the root of the lungs. Neither does its absence afford any positive conclusions on the other side. In the succeeding part of this volume a dissection will be related, in which that gland was a scirrhous mass, whilst the urine was remarkably pale and loaded with albumen, and totally devoid of sediment of any kind * ; so uncertain are what we call pathognomic signs ; and so much safer is it to determine from all the appearances collected together, than from any single symptom, however important.

In the early stage of the disorder medical treatment does a great deal, principally by means of diuretics ; and squill is by far the most powerful of them. This drug gives out its virtues so perfectly to different menstrua, as to make the form of its exhibition in that respect a matter of indifference. But a solution of it is much more accurately and easily dosed than the powder, and probably admits of a more ready absorption. A minute attention to its dose is likewise of great consequence. It never operates so favourably, as when it is given in the fullest quantity which the patient can bear without sickness. Indeed, that excellent practical writer, Van Swieten, as well as Dr. Cullen, considered some degree of nausea as proper for securing its diuretic effect. But few persons can be brought to submit to this for several days in succes-

* Chap. VII. Case V.

sion; and it appears to be an unnecessary piece of severity, particularly as a risk must thus sometimes be incurred of producing full vomiting, which greatly prevents its future use as a diuretic. It is therefore proper to begin with a dose of the vinegar or tincture of squill, so small as not to incur any reasonable chance of sickness, and to increase the quantity gradually, till either the desired effect takes place, or some degree of nausea. Just under this point it should be continued, till it operates favourably, which will often be in a few days. In this manner it may be exhibited three times daily, and commencing with thirty drops the quantity may be increased to forty or fifty.

The mistura ammoniaci and spiritus ætheris nitrici seem to assist its operation.

With the foregoing cautions, the squill will be found to produce very great effects. The urine becomes pale and copious under its use; proportional relief is obtained in the breathing and in the diffused swellings; and it seldom either purges or palls the appetite, as it is justly accused of doing under other circumstances. Frequent repetition only, and the increasing strength of the original malady, impair its action ; and if we look for any great effect from it in removing the visceral obstructions, we shall undoubtedly be disappointed.

In recommending this article, I am glad not to introduce any novelty. The materia medica is already loaded with powerful instruments, which rather want precision in their direction than any increase to their number. The squill is one of these. Its effects on the system are always powerful, frequently beneficial. But it is too indiscriminately employed, and often rather with a fortunate conjecture, than under any precise laws. The appearances, in short, that should regulate its exhibition, are certainly not even yet, after the experience of so many ages, understood as they ought to be. Why else have we to lament, I will not say, its occasional want of success, (for that must always be expected,) but the injury which it sometimes does to the digestive organs, and the rapidity with which the system sinks under its use ? No medicine ever aggravated the complaint for which it was directed, but by some mistake in the prescriber. The rules for its employment have been misapplied, or, such are the manifold imperfections of our art, have never been agreed upon even by the most skilful practitioners. It apologizes for all errors, to atttribute these bad effects to an idiosyncracy, and to state them not to be discoverable but by experiment in each individual. I should hope that in the instance alluded to they are rather the result of the form which the disease assumes, and which is capable of being denoted by its external signs.

The colchicum is probably suited to the same occasions as the squill. But I have not had much experience of it.

In removing glandular obstructions, the preparations of mercury are considered to hold a principal rank. Its assistance as a diuretic is undoubtedly not inconsiderable. For when the squill does not act entirely as could be wished, the addition of a grain or two of the submuriate of mercury, every night, is frequently followed by a great flow of urine, at the same time that the salivary glands are affected. As to any further aid from it, our expectations ought to be re-

strained by the recollection of many discouraging circumstances connected with the
advanced age and free habits of the suf-
ferers, and of the extensive havoc we often
meet with on dissection. There are obstructions in the liver, even attended by
ascites, which courses of mercury remove;
but on the scirrhous or tuberculated state of
that gland, a frequent cause of dropsy in
this country, I have seldom seen it make
any impression. It would be somewhat in
its favour to add, that it is universally safe.
I dare not assert this; since I have seen in
such instances the mercurial habit superadded by continued salivation, and thus the
disorder become more complicated and
more speedily fatal.

Squills having answered so well as a diuretic in the circumstances before described,
my experience of the digitalis is very limited in them, and does not entitle me to
say any thing decided respecting it.

These patients bear purging badly; and
the operation seldom carries off much water.

Tonics in any stage uniformly do harm,
and reproduce the swellings.

CHAPTER V.

OF DROPSIES, IN WHICH THE URINE IS COAGULABLE BY HEAT.

THE presence of serum in the urine, as discovered by the application of heat, is not entirely confined to dropsies. It certainly cannot be considered as a common occurrence in other diseases, much less in health; but sometimes, where without any effusions the emaciation has been greater than could be accounted for by the obvious symptoms, I have suspected that this process was taking place, and in two instances have detected it, though in a very slight degree. In one of these we found on dissection an extensive scirrhus of the stomach near the pylorus; in the other there had been a large hæmorrhage from the nose, succeeded

by the most extreme dejection of spirits
and loss of strength. I have likewise some
suspicions that the excessive use of the al-
kalies and magnesia disposes the serum of
the blood to pass off by the kidneys. This
symptom is, however, rarely found to exist,
perhaps never, in any considerable degree,
but as a sign of some dropsy either forming
or already formed. These are the anasarca,
hydrothorax, ascites and hydrocephalus,
with their various combinations. Many
cases indeed are very imperfectly described
by either of these terms singly, and are
rather a general dropsy, involving the cellular membrane extensively, and one or
more of the large cavities likewise. For
these there is no appropriate title in our
books of nosology; but as the anasarca is
their most obvious and early symptom, and
the existence of the internal accumulation
is often more or less doubtful, I have
arranged them with the former. The anasarca strictly speaking, and for any long
period, is comparatively rare.

The continuance of this disease is generally followed by a depravation of the whole
habit, and by that sallow transparency of

G

complexion which cannot fail to strike even an inexperienced observer. There are many cases, in which these alarming signs give their character to the œdematous swellings, from their very commencement, and in which the patients have been pronounced to be in a cachexy, even before the dropsy has been completely formed. This state, although called a species of anasarca, has appeared to me to be entitled to a separate consideration in the present enquiry. It is very apt to terminate in universal effusions, and often in old subjects in an hydrothorax. Petechiæ are sometimes superadded to it; and it is then not easily distinguishable, if indeed it be at all different, from the land-scurvy.

CHAPTER VI.

OF THE ANASARCA AND GENERAL DROPSY, IN WHICH THE URINE IS COAGULABLE BY HEAT.

THE dropsy diffused through the cellular membrane, and in its progress usually involving the large cavities likewise, is a very common form of the disease. Its exciting causes are sometimes sufficiently remarkable, and where they can be readily ascertained, constitute a natural and useful distinction, of which I have availed myself in arranging the cases contained in this chapter.

One of these causes is scarlatina, which operates to a great extent in certain seasons; another is courses of mercury imprudently conducted, and perhaps aided by cold; a

G 2

third the drinking of cold water, when heated ; and I have reserved a fourth section for those cases, in which the exciting cause was not very obvious nor precise, but appeared connected with different circumstances of fatigue, cold, the use of strong liquors, visceral disease, or the injudicious employment of tonics.

In the histories themselves the general character of the urine is given, and the extent of its coagulation by heat. The occasional experiments, which I have tried with other chemical tests, are to prevent the necessity of repetition, placed together. I lament, undoubtedly, that they are so few and so limited, because the discharge of albumen by this unusual channel might probably be much illustrated, by ascertaining whether any saline matters were present, that particularly favoured its solution. The complicated nature of that fluid, at all times, but especially in disease, seems to surround the subject with difficulties.

SECTION I.

Cases of Anasarca, &c. after Scarlatina, with a Dissection. — Remarks.

CASE I.

E. Hammet, ætat. 42, Hospital, June, 1798, had been confined by scarlatina five months since, and three weeks afterwards had become dropsical. At the time of her admission she had an ascites, very universal anasarca, great feebleness and frequency of pulse, with general weakness and a bad appetite.

The urine was nearly natural in colour and quantity. On being subjected to heat the whole fluid was rendered uniformly opaque at 160°, and soon deposited a considerable coagulum.

Squills, the bitter alkaline infusion, crystals of tartar, and many other diuretics and purgatives, were exhibited without effect. Her apparent loss of tone induced me to try bark and steel, both with and without eva-

cuants ; but they aggravated the symptoms.
At length scarifications of the legs were employed, and there was much discharge from
the wounds. This fluid gave no precipitate
even at boiling heat, and very little by the
addition of nitrous acid. The œdema was
not permanently lessened by these means;
but in two or three weeks a severe erysipelas
of the lower extremities followed, and gangrenous spots, with a total failure of strength.
In this dangerous state it was necessary to
give bark and port wine very largely. These
not only succeeded in stopping the erysipelas, but encouraged such a flow of urine and
discharge from the legs, as speedily unloaded her. The urine in this increased
quantity contained a less proportion of serum ; and greater heat was required for its
precipitation. Discontinuing the bark too
soon, she became again somewhat œdematous, the urine altering in the same proportion ; and it was only by returning to a
long and regular course of that medicine,
that she perfectly recovered.

CASE II.

R. D. ætat. 10, just recovered from an attack of scarlatina, so slight, that he had been hardly kept one day from school, complained of pain on the outside of the right leg, somewhat above the ancle. The part was very hot, difficult to be moved, slightly swelled as if from rheumatism, and did not retain the impression of the finger. This seemed to be the complaint, which his friends noticed most. I observed besides a quick and feverish pulse, with a bloated abdomen, pale purple lips, languor and shortness of breathing. The night before, he had been awakened by some spasm on his chest, and cough. His urine on examination proved to be scanty, and very serous.

A few mild purges reduced his fever, and brought him into a state in which he bore the cinchona well. The urine then cleared, and he recovered.

CASE III.

M. J. ætat. 10, anasarca; ascites; palpitations of the heart, dyspnœa, excessive

anguor ; urine pale, not scanty, nor depositing any sediment, but greatly loaded
with serum.

These symptoms had succeeded a mild
scarlatina about ten days before. Bark
had produced a tightness of the chest;
and under the use of calomel, squill, and
other diuretics, there was a rapid increase
of all the bad signs. Particularly, the exhibition of two grains of calomel, every
night, had been followed by great debility
and frequent retching.

I directed two drachms of the infusum
digitalis every day, which restored her
speedily.

CASE IV.

J. E. ætat. 12, had recovered from scarlatina about three weeks, when he became
suddenly dropsical. There was an ascites
and very universal anasarca, the scrotum
particularly being enormously distended. I
found his urine so overloaded, as to resemble serum of the blood three or four times

diluted with water. It was high-coloured, and contained a bloody sediment.

Two drachms of the infusum of digitalis, every eight hours, soon removed his swellings, whilst the urine immediately became more diluted, and in a short time quite natural. Let me add once for all, that in the instances of cure by digitalis, this improvement of the urinary discharge is simultaneous with a relief of the other symptoms, is certainly not subsequent to them, but always amongst the earliest good signs. This child, however, continued feeble, and although the dropsy did not return, yet on again applying the test of heat to the urine, whilst he was continuing that remedy, it became quite opaque at boiling heat.

The Peruvian bark soon corrected this appearance; and he regained strength rapidly.

CASE V.

E. W. ætat. 3, sister of the child, whose recovery is related under the article hydrocephalus, lay ill of scarlatina at the same time, and when I visited him, was quite anasarcous.

The urine was turbid even when made, speedily deposited a dark bloody sediment, and was overloaded with serum.

The sediment did not in this and the other instances disappear by a slight heat, as it would have done if it had been of the branny kind, but gave a brown tinge to the coagulum.

The infusion of digitalis carried off these symptoms; and she required some Peruvian bark for the re-establishment of her appetite and strength.

CASE VI.

F. M. ætat. 7, about three weeks after a slight attack of scarlatina, began to swell, and had been purged by medicines, of which calomel formed a principal ingredient, in consequence of which his symptoms increased.

I found him with the legs slightly swelled, abdomen considerably; and he could not lie down in bed. His urine was very scanty, foul when made, and soon deposited something that appeared to be lymph, and likewise a bloody mucus. Much under boiling heat, it grew very opaque, and exhaled a most fœtid odour.

Small doses of digitalis rendered him service; and he then took Peruvian bark with great advantage.

CASE VII.

E. C. ætat. 8, in the fifth week after a mild scarlatina became dropsical. During the exhibition of mercurial purges, the swellings of the extremities had been reduced. But a very considerable ascites remained, with a bloated pale complexion, stiffness of the knees, great feebleness, a quick pulse, and much pain between the eye-brows. Her urine was scanty, foul, quite discoloured with blood, and greatly loaded with albumen.

I considered this child as on the verge of an hydrocephalus; but most of her bad symptoms disappeared in a few days under the use of the fox-glove; the ascites continued longer, and was not finally removed till she took the Peruvian bark.

CASE VIII.

L. D. ætat. 8, became generally bloated and swelled, in the abdomen particularly, about ten days after the disappearance of the scarlatinous eruption.

I found his urine rather scanty and pale, very slightly changed by boiling heat, and giving some coagulum on the application of the nitrous acid. On standing, it deposited a loose bloody sediment.

This child had taken no medicine at any period of the disease.

Very small doses of digitalis every way unloaded him, but during its continuance, greater symptoms of feebleness came on without swelling; and the urine again precipitated something by heat.

The cinchona in substance restored him speedily.

CASE IX.

J. N. ætat. 16, passed through a very mild attack of scarlatina, and about a month after, as if from a recent cold, became slightly anasarcous in the extremities, and affected with some shortness of breathing.

His medical attendant very judiciously gave him the fox-glove, which much relieved him. At this period, however, I was consulted, and finding that the urine was very slightly discoloured by heat, and as little by nitrous acid, (which is often the case after that remedy has done its office,) and that his pulse was quick and feeble, I ordered the cinchona, in great hopes that all stricture of the chest was removed. The contrary proved to be the fact; and I was obliged to have recourse to small doses of tincture of digitalis, under which plan he soon recovered.

CASE X.

Sarah Ellicot, ætat. 30, was brought into the Devon and Exeter Hospital, 1800, in a state of great distress, labouring under universal anasarca, and an erysipelatous inflammation of the lower extremities, with much discharge, and deep sloughs on the hips and sacrum.

The urine coagulated, although not to the extent sometimes observed; and it flowed freely, as I have often noticed it to do, whenever much serum is discharged from the legs.

She had the remains of a florid sanguine temperament, and had been in good health till about two months before, when a fever with great redness of the face and extremities attacked her; soon after which she had become dropsical, and affected likewise with stricture of the chest, cough, and pain under the left breast. All her present symptoms demanded the cinchona, which she took in very large doses, and with great advantage. She was quite in-

undated with the discharges from the legs
and the increased flow of urine. The erysipelas disappeared, and, shortly after, all
vestiges of dropsy. But the sloughs above
mentioned had penetrated deeper than we
hoped; the bones became carious, and
about two months after, she died exhausted, the anasarca never having returned.

It was not uninteresting for me to ascertain by dissection the state of the internal
parts, and particularly the kidneys; not,
indeed, that I suspected any thing more
than a disordered secretion from that
gland; but that it is always satisfactory
to leave nothing to conjecture, on subjects
where ocular demonstration is to be obtained.

The kidneys were rather soft and flaccid,
and more loaded with fat than could have
been supposed after so long an illness,
but in other respects quite natural. There
was no morbid appearance in any other
viscera of the abdomen.

The pleura of the left lung bore marks of
inflammation, more severe than the common adhesive; for small flakes and granula

of coagulated lymph covered it in several parts, principally in a spot answering to the seat of the pain during life ; and that membrane was separated from the body of the lung for about the size of a shilling, by a very small deposition of pus.   Opposite the same spot the pleura costalis was inflamed.   In other respects the substance of the thoracic viscera was sound, and there was no unusual quantity of water in the cavities.

———

The bloody sediment observed in the urine, in no less than five of these ten cases, is well worthy of notice, as indicating how nearly the other remarkable character of it is allied to a true hæmorrhage. It is not quite peculiar to the scarlatinous dropsy, nor to the early age at which that fever usually occurs ; as will be seen in the succeeding pages.   I have thought it to be hastened and encouraged by the use of mercury.   That this sediment does actually derive its colour from the presence of red blood, is evinced by its appearance, which can hardly deceive, by its being so speedily deposited, and by its remaining undissolved when heat is again applied. It has not been wholly overlooked by authors.

Von Rosenstein states, that the urine is mixed with blood in some patients, when the body swells after scarlatina. * Burserius describes it as *turbida et fusca, et quandoque omnino suppressa;* and adds in a note, that it has been found to resemble in colour water, in which flesh had been washed. †

The dissection in case X. possesses some value. Practitioners have usually thought themselves justified in supposing the serous membranes to be relaxed only, and discharging too much fluid from their numerous exhalants. We here find the pleura to be inflamed, and even partially suppurated.

Burserius notices the presence of internal inflammation, particularly peripneumony, in the scarlatinous œdema, and adds,

* See Von Rosenstein on the Diseases of Children. *Sparrman's Translation, p.* 166.
† Burserius' Institutes, vol. 2d, p. 80.

H

that this opinion of its nature has been confirmed by dissection, and by the great advantages derived from blood-letting. He draws, however, a distinction between the *œdema calidum* and *frigidum*, which appears to me not perfectly correct. The former of these, known by an increased temperature, florid colour, and hardness, of the parts affected, he considers to be an inflammatory state, and curable by antiphlogistics ; whilst the latter, a pale and cold œdema, is usually without fever, and to be treated like a common anasarca.* I have not made experiments on the blood of persons so attacked, because I have found them curable by milder means ; but if there is any analogy between this and other dropsies, the cold and soft œdema is by no means inconsistent with great inflammation of the habit.

Digitalis is its sovereign remedy. Dr. Withering has made this assertion without reserve respecting the scarlatinous anasarca. †   Applied to that form of the dis-

---

* Burserius' Institutes, vol. 2d, p. 81.
† Withering's Account of the Fox-glove, p. 25.

ease which we are now considering, it is
strictly correct. I know of no instance
where digitalis has failed, when properly
exhibited; and I add, without fear of
contradiction, that it is equal to almost
every emergency, short of that destruction
of parts, which admits of no cure. But I
must again request the reader, to bear in
his mind the exception to the general character of such cases, contained in the beginning of the second chapter, and the
failure of digitalis in that instance. *

SECTION II.

*Of the Anasarca, &c. from Mercury, with
Dissections and Remarks.*

CASE I.

L. G. ætat. 25, 1806, had been, when
he consulted me, just undergoing a mercu-

* Page 5.

rial course of two months' continuance for a
venereal complaint; during which he was
become universally and rather suddenly
anasarcous.

The urine was scanty, high-coloured, and
deposited a branny and lateritious sediment.   It was much loaded with serum.
He besides complained of cough and pain
in his left side.   Some blood was on this
account taken from the arm, and found
watery, but inflamed.   Crystals of tartar
were then prescribed in large doses, and
the legs directed to be scarified.   But with
unusual severity the surgeon made several
scarifications of four inches in length on
each leg.   I expected nothing better than
a sphacelus.   By fomentations, however,
the inflammation was restrained; and the
discharge was so excessive as to pass
through the patient's bed repeatedly upon
the floor every day.   To support this, he
soon required a very cordial treatment,
both bark and port wine, and under that
plan was quite restored.

CASE II.

H. G. ætat. 12, was suspected by her parents to have worms, and took by their direction some doses of an empirical medicine, containing calomel. Her gums were not observed to be affected; neither was she much purged; but very soon after, and without any other assignable cause, she became almost suddenly œdematous in every part of her body; an ascites speedily followed; and the pain in her left side, and dyspnœa on motion, made me suspect the thorax likewise.

I found her urine to be very pale, speedily putrefying, and loaded with a white sediment and flakes, part of which, from its being insoluble by heat, I considered to be lymph. The clear fluid did not much alter before boiling heat; but then became thick and ropy, and on the slightest evaporation was converted into a mass nearly gelatinous in appearance.

I tried digitalis with considerable confidence in this instance; and the immediate result showed that I had fixed rightly. The urine in a few days was increased in quantity, and its coagulum much lessened. The swellings began to diminish; but being removed into the country, she took larger doses of the tincture of digitalis than were directed, and died suddenly, the anasarca and ascites having previously almost disappeared.

CASE III.

L. N. ætat. 50, 1804, had been labouring for more than three years under constitutional symptoms of the lues venerea, and had used repeated courses of mercury for many months together, from which his general health suffered extremely. I considered the venereal taint to be eradicated, and that his symptoms were attributable to mercury, a great dejection of mind, a sallow countenance, perpetual diarrhœa, pains in the joints, restless nights, no sleep being obtained but by large doses of opium, a rapid pulse, considerable anasarca, and urine loaded with

serum. The anasarca had been very gradual in its appearance. Sarsaparilla and
mezereon he tried largely without effect.
Under the use of one drachm of nitrous
acid daily, for two months, he gained
strength, and lost his pains ; but the swellings and loaded urine still continued. He
bore no tonics, and seemed to be still less a
subject for evacuations.

As he lived at a distance of more than
ten miles from me, I saw him but seldom.
In my absence the attendant apothecary
drew a few ounces of blood from his arm,
on account of a violent pain at the pit of
the stomach, from which he had long suffered in some degree, with greater severity
only a few hours.

To my surprize, when I visited him the
next day, I found the blood completely inflamed. The serum exactly resembled run-
net whey in colour and appearance, and the
small coagulum which swam in the midst
was covered with a thin, white, extremely
firm, crust, cupped to little more than the
size of a half crown. The serum coagulated strongly by heat. Whoever had been

witness to this state of the blood, must have been convinced that it was not the process of a day. I was, however, fearful, considering all the circumstances, of evacuating him further, and he soon afterwards died.

CASE IV.

Robert Mock, ætat. 50, a sailor, was admitted into the Hospital, 1809, partly on account of a severe sloughing ulcer of the left leg, the tibia of which was enlarged. His constitutional symptoms likewise were very formidable; a general sallowness, great dejection of spirits, and loss of muscular strength, a slight but tense œdema of the lower extremities, a very chorded pulse, a moist clean tongue, thirst, total loss of appetite, and frequent vomiting, particularly of aperient medicines. He had neither cough nor orthopnœa. The urinary discharge amounted to about three quarts in twenty-four hours, the principal part being made in the night. It was very pale and clear, deposited no sediment, retained for many days its quality of reddening infusion of litmus, and continued long free from any apparent putrefaction. It became opaque at 160° of heat, and soon deposited large and firm flakes. From four ounces of clear urine placed in a phial before the fire for a few minutes, were obtained forty grains of a solid coagulum, which was in the proportion of two ounces to the quantity of urine discharged daily. It lost by a very moderate desiccation only one-fourth part of its weight.

He was very uniform in his statement, that the ulcer had originated, more than twenty years before, in the sting of an insect in North America. For its cure he had been admitted into many hospitals in this country without effect; and had undergone several salivations, partly for syphilitic complaints, of which he had been the repeated victim. One very long course of mercury he had suffered about twelve months before, and during it some degree of anasarca had come on, which for many

months affected only the sound leg, afterwards both.   Lately he had been taking
Peruvian bark with an aggravation of his
symptoms.

The ulcer was soon reduced to nearly an
healing state, by the use of the fermenting
cataplasm; but with no relief to his constitution.   The oedema in a few days partly
quitted the limbs before affected, and spread
to the covering of the abdomen and thorax
and to the arms; or it was rather a pale
tense tumour, hardly retaining the impression of the finger, and in some slight degree sore to the touch.

Aperient medicines were rendered inadmissible by an extreme irritability of the
stomach, and a most painful prolapsus.
Of the tincture of foxglove not more than
two or three drops could be borne without
vomiting.   Blood drawn to the amount of
sixteen ounces was very much inflamed,
and cupped, and not watery; the serum
of a whey colour.   He bore the operation
well, and the pulse was somewhat reduced.
For a day or two after the urine gave very
little precipitate by heat, but it gradually

resumed its former character. From the
cold weather of January he suffered extremely, not being able to obtain the least
sensation of warmth. A dry cough likewise took place, with some stricture upon
the chest, and excruciating pain darting
from the sternum to the back quite through
the region of the heart. A tendency to
deliquium was likewise observed on raising
himself in bed ; but he could lie down horizontally. The pulse was about eighty,
strong and hard, but by no means interrupted. It was impossible not to conclude
that the membranes surrounding the heart
were inflamed. Besides the use of blisters,
a large venæ-section was instantly directed ;
and he lost nearly thirty ounces of blood,
before there was the least reduction of the
hardness of the pulse. At the end of that
operation it became nearly natural, and the
pain wholly subsided. The blood, though
only trickling from the orifice, on account
of the difficulty which the œdema of the
arm presented, was in the highest degree
inflamed and cupped. The relief, however, was only temporary ; and his bodily

weakness, as well as the anasarca, certainly
increased. Several returns of pain and
stricture, though in less degree, rendered
bleeding again necessary. He lost in about
a month somewhat more than an hundred
ounces of blood, always in a very inflamed
state, and always with present relief, although not so direct a diminution of the
quantity of serum in the urine. The recurrence of his bad symptoms, and a
greater softness of the œdema said to indicate digitalis, induced me again to have
recourse to it. He now bore it in doses or
twenty drops every eight hours ; but it had
no beneficial effect upon him, notwithstanding that it produced a great retardation of the pulse, 'and the feelings peculiar
to its poisonous action. Some diarrhœa
ensued, which remained with him to his
death. His urine became gradually less
serous, and more putrescent. He grew
feebler, at last tympanitic, and had sloughs
on his hips and sacrum. In this way he
terminated a most miserable existence.

On opening the body, we found, on the
right side of the thorax, twelve ounces of

serum, in which were some floating membranes ; the pleura in several parts inflamed,
and covered with exudations of lymph ;
the left side nearly in the same state, the
fluid about ten ounces : the lungs sound,
but rather overloaded with blood in the
posterior part, and at their roots ; the pericardium, both the investing membrane and
its duplicature, thickened and inflamed,
and in many places quite woolly, with
flakes of lymph adhering to it, particularly
about the origin of the great artery ; in
the cavity three ounces of a turbid whitish
fluid ; the heart very large, pale and firm,
and three or four ossified spots in the
inner membrane of the aorta.

In the abdomen, the stomach was greatly
distended with air ; the omentum rather
thickened ; the peritoneal coverings of the
spleen and liver dull and slightly inflamed,
particularly that of the former, which was
likewise connected by adhesions to the surrounding parts ; the latter of these glands
rather firmer than ordinary ; the kidneys
likewise unusually firm ; in the left, one
very small hydatid, in the right two ; more

than an ounce of fluid in each lateral ventricle of the brain.

The cellular membrane of the trunk and
extremities was every where loaded with a
coagulated semi-transparent effusion, which
gave an unusual resistance to the knife.
This was particularly the case in the pa-
rieties of the abdomen, and in the loins,
and certainly explained the tension and
soreness to the touch not common in anasarca. The fluid which drained off from
the incisions was very glutinous, and on
exposure to air for some time formed into
an apparently gelatinous substance, which,
on being heated, separated into a solid
lymph and thin fluid. The serum of the
pericardium coagulated strongly by heat ;
that from the thorax and abdomen in a
less degree, and the water of the ventricles of the brain was the most diluted,
though still coagulating to an unusual
extent.

In the two former of these cases the attack was rather sudden, and probably aided by cold or some other cause of inflammation. The latter are specimens of a true mercurial habit, slowly forming, distinguished in their advanced stage by a most unconquerable buffiness of the blood, and an unusual colour even of the serum. They perhaps belong rather to the article, cachexy ; but I preferred placing them in this section on account of the identity of the exciting cause, and for the purpose of better illustrating the action of this mineral. No one can contemplate these remarkable characters of the blood, the dry cough and pains in the side, the thickened membranes and turbid fluid discovered on dissection, and particularly the spontaneous coagulation of the fluid taken from the cellular membrane, without forming conclusions favourable to the doctrine of an inflammation induced by mercurial courses, and of the great risk of that inflammation fixing internally. It is likewise a circumstance of some importance, that the urinary discharge so often alluded to, which carries with it the suspicion of debility, may be united with an ex-

cessive arterial action in no ordinary degree,
and is sometimes relieved by the same
means. There are, however, exceptions to
this coagulable state of the urine *, which
are probably to be attributed to the mercury passing off rapidly by the bowels, and
thus leaving the constitution weakened
rather than inflamed.

The five following cases are added, not
as examples of a complete mercurial dropsy,
but to show of what nature those slighter
swellings of the extremities are, which often
follow the use of mercury in certain constitutions : but I willingly avail myself of an
opportunity of recording the fifth in particular, and the annexed dissection, as
containing the history of a malady not yet
sufficiently noticed by physicians.

CASE I.

A young woman from Jamaica had been

* Pages 21 and 22.

undergoing in that island repeated salivations for the yellow fever, and its subsequent
obstructions. Her health had been completely shaken by these causes. She remained affected with darting pains through
her right side, a great deal of dyspnœa on
motion, puffy, œdematous, irregularly shift-
ing, swellings of the ancles, knees, and other
joints, and an urine giving a coagulum under the boiling heat.

I had many reasons connected with the
history of her complaint, for attributing
these circumstances to mercury; and they
certainly indicated a state quite unfit for
such an exhibition of that mineral, as the
pains of the liver seemed to require.

CASE II.

R. L. ætat. 30, persisted in the use of
mercurial friction, for pains of the joints
undoubtedly aggravated by mercury. One
of his legs became œdematous, and the urine
slightly coagulated by heat. He readily
gave up his former plan, and by change of
air and sarsaparilla was restored.

I

CASE III.

R. M. ætat. 50, burst an internal abscess, that had been connected with pain in the region of the spleen. The pus discharged itself upwards and downwards; and suspicious sputa with cough remained. Mercurials were ordered by the attending practitioner; but his gums became shortly affected, and his legs at the same time œdematous.

The urine examined at that period was found somewhat impregnated with serum.

The sputa likewise assumed a form more decidedly purulent.

On the discontinuance of the mercury, the urine gradually improved.

CASE IV.

G. H. ætat. 30, was recommended to the coast of Devonshire on account of a cough and spitting of blood. Severe bilious symptoms came on during his residence there, with jaundice, an apparent induration of the right side, and a very remarkable dyspnœa.

Two grains of calomel were exhibited every night with great advantage, in respect to these symptoms, and particularly his respiration. But at the end of a week his legs swelled, and the urine on examination was found partially to coagulate.

CASE V.

G. Hatswell, ætat. 35, Hospital, 1811, of a scrophulous habit, and blind in his right eye, in consequence of that taint, was put under a mercurial course on account of a diarrhœa, the circumstances of which I shall presently describe. His gums were with difficulty affected; he grew weak; and his legs began to swell. The urine examined at this time became opaque considerably under the boiling heat, which had been particularly ascertained not to be the fact previous to the exhibition of mercury; and after the discontinuance of that mineral for a fortnight or three weeks, some œdema still remaining, this appearance gradually lessened, although it never entirely ceased.

The diarrhœa, for which such a course had been prescribed, was of a remarkable kind, consisting of discharges which nearly resembled yeast in colour, fluidity, and effervescence. They were likewise extremely copious, and followed by the most excessive sinking. He suffered altogether more from flatulency, dyspepsia, and dejection of spirits, than from any precise pain; sometimes, however, he complained of stitches in his left side, to which he had been subject in consequence of a strain and hæmoptoe four years before; and when questioned would acknowledge an obscure uneasiness and fulness towards the lower part of the abdomen, on the right side. This I apprehend increased latterly.

He had been ill several months, and continued to emaciate and grow feebler, till he was reduced to a mere skeleton. Cough and purulent expectoration were amongst his last symptoms.

The suspicion of a liver disease, which most of us perhaps are too willing to entertain, induced me to put him under the influence of mercury. In a saline form, this mineral greatly disagreed with him. A small quantity of pilulæ hydrargyri, guarded by large doses of opium, with some difficulty affected his gums; and certainly at the same time the discharges became more solid, and coloured with green bile. But he had not firmness enough for such a course; the diarrhœa returned; and he again lost ground rapidly.

Astringents greatly bloated and oppressed him. Nothing but tincture of opium at all palliated his complaints; and under the use of it, his diarrhœa subsided for three weeks before his death. Two months preceding this event, he had become an out-patient; and I therefore cannot speak precisely with regard to several of his latter symptoms, particularly the presence of blood or pus in his discharges.

The examination of the body baffled all our conjectures. The liver was natural both in size and structure, and the gall-bladder full of a yellow healthy bile. But on tracing the intestines, we found the cæcum and its appendix, with some of the neighbouring parts, involved in a mass of scrophulous adhesions, which, when taken out and dissected at leisure, presented the following appearances. The disease began about two inches above the termination of the ileum. Its inner membrane was, to the extent of a crown-piece, covered with spots of lymph; and there were two or three small ulcers. The whole of the inner membrane of the cæcum was completely destroyed by ulceration, and its other coats much thickened; the beginning of the colon in the same state, for five or six inches further nearly healthy, and then again for a short space thickened and ulcerated, in a spot where by a sort of unusual course of the intestine it had doubled down upon the cæcum, and was involved in the same mass of adhesions. The remaining part of the great intestines appeared to be sound; but we did not make any minute examination of it; the glands of the mesocolon were enlarged; the kidneys remarkably loaded with blood as if injected; the lungs were full of tubercles partially suppurated.

I apprehend a slight degree of this disease

16

to be not unusual.   I have seen four cases of
it to an extraordinary extent, where the discharges by stool greatly resembled yeast in
their appearance, and in one instance were
nearly raised by their effervescence over the
sides of the vessel.   All the patients had
this in common, that they died extremely
emaciated, and after a most tedious lingering.   Their depression of spirits was excessive; their sinking after these discharges
dreadful, with a sensation as if the whole
body were coming out; frequently they
expected not to survive them.   In all there
was much flatulency, and in some a croak-
ing noise of air, apparently seated in the
ascending arch of the colon, and sometimes
producing such a projection there, as almost to give suspicion of a ventral hernia.
Pain they did not suffer in proportion to
their other symptoms.   One of them had
been subject to hæmorrhoids, and prolapsus
ani.   Mercury, even by friction, could not
be brought to affect the gums of any but
the subject of the present case, and there
without any advantage; and the debilitating effects of the saline preparations of
that mineral were very great.

Writers describe this remarkable complaint imperfectly; and when they notice the occurrence of yeasty discharges, they generally seem to refer them to an obstruction of the liver exclusively. But many circumstances, particularly the preceding dissection, prove the large intestines to be much engaged in this disorder. And although it is possible that vitiated secretions from the upper part of the alimentary canal, and food imperfectly converted, may be the primary cause of such excoriations of the lower bowels, as acrid bile is in the dysentery of the East, yet it is no small point, to be satisfied, that the liver is not organically unsound, that mercury is injurious, that deobstruents are not called for. I consider opiates as the most likely to render benefit, with small doses of ipecacuanha, and probably a course of the Bath waters.

The cœliaca passio of Aretæus resembles it in many points. *

* Aretæus de morbus diuturnis, lib. 2d, chap. 7th.

SECTION III.

Of the Anasarca, &c. from drinking cold Water, when heated and fatigued.

CASE I.

R. E. ætat. 50, 1801, in the evening after returning from work, having been much exposed to heat, and drank cold water in that state, was attacked with febrile symptoms, attended by pain of his left side, and inability of lying on it. In two or three days he became universally anasarcous.

I was consulted for him three weeks afterwards, and found that his urine was both scanty, and much overloaded with serum. There was a very strong and full pulse, a total loss of appetite, and a rotten taste in the mouth, with a dry costive habit.

He had been taking purges of jalap and cream of tartar occasionally, with some advantage. I continued the cream of tartar principally in large doses; and the urine

flowing with much freedom, he soon recovered complete health, under the use of
Peruvian bark.

CASE II.

William Rowe, a stout and large man,
ætat. 35, Hospital, 1809; very extensive
anasarca; bloated and sallow countenance;
pulse 90, quick, chorded, redoubling; urine
coagulating at a low heat, when recent,
reddening infusion of litmus, but soon putrefying; there was no ascites, nor, as far
as we could judge from the total absence of
cough and orthopnœa, any probability of
hydrothorax.

He attributed the attack to drinking a
large quantity of cold water when heated,
and fatigued by labour in the harvest,
more than twelve months before. He was
the same evening seized with rigors, but
no local pain, and soon became universally
anasarcous.

Squills had little or no effect on the swellings. His pulse continued very chorded;
and he complained of a throbbing in differ-

ent parts, particularly his head with a kind
of confusion of thought. These symptoms
made me think venæ-section, however unusual in dropsy, advisable. The blood
drawn was watery, but covered with a remarkably thick and firm buff; and he was
much relieved by the loss of about ten
ounces.

I then directed daily large doses of crystals of tartar, under which plan the inflammatory symptoms soon left him; the swellings still further subsided; and he began to
feel a vertigo, and a numbness of his limbs,
aggravated by purging. The urine in this
state was still coagulable, although by a
greater heat and less firmly. By large doses
of bark this appearance was removed in a
fortnight or three weeks; and he entirely recovered, a painful ulcer in his leg of some
weeks continuance healing at the same time.
It is probable that this drain had acted very
beneficially in preventing some determination to the internal parts.

Case II. is an example of a very severe and long continued inflammation of the blood, not connected with any corresponding affection of the internal parts. Can we suppose it possible, that such a disposition as this should be merely general? Or, is the cellular membrane in these instances the seat of an obscure inflammatory process, in which the exhalant arteries are too active, and secrete a fluid every way unfit for its purposes?

SECTION IV.

Cases of Anasarca, &c. from Cold, Intemperance, &c. — Remarks.

CASE I.

W. L. ætat. 60, a very robust man, had noticed, about a fortnight before I was called to him, a swelling of one leg without any precise constitutional complaint. In that state he attended the funeral of a neighbour, was much exposed to cold and rain, and, as I was informed, drank freely of some strong liquors. An universal anasarca succeeded in a very few days.

I observed considerable suppressed cough, pain at the pit of the stomach, and some orthopnœa, with many marks of an inflamed chest, particularly great protrusion of the abdomen in breathing, and a proportional difficulty of elevating the ribs; pulse 90, quick, hard. The anasarcous swellings were by far the greatest, I ever witnessed. The urine was very scanty and foul, with a red sediment; and on being heated it thickened into a white and opaque mass, which soon became nearly solid. He had been scarified in the legs and scrotum, before I visited him. The wounds were now inflaming with great pain; and an erysipelas extended from them almost over the whole body. These complicated complaints proved fatal to him in a few days. I never saw a dropsy run so rapid a course, nor stronger signs of pleuritic inflammation joined to it. The state of the scarified parts, which were becoming rapidly gangrenous, deterred me, perhaps not with sufficient reason, from adopting those active measures which could alone at any time have saved his life.

CASE II.

H. R. ætat. 70, 1806, a washer-woman, robust and of a ruddy complexion, had an universal anasarca, some cough, soreness of the chest and dyspnœa, with a quick and hard pulse; urine pale and apparently thin, becoming quite opaque at 160°, depositing no sediment, remaining for a long time free from putrefaction, and for more than a week reddening litmus paper. The quantity made was between one and two quarts daily; and the coagulum, obtained from one quart placed before the fire for a few minutes, amounted to ten drachms, which lost by moderate desiccation nearly half its weight.

She had been attacked about a month before with a swelling of one leg, in the groin of which there was an enlarged lymphatic gland. A legitimate dropsy speedily followed, all which she attributed to cold, and the fatiguing posture necessary in her employment.

I directed blisters to the chest, and some
purgatives, consisting of jalap and crystals
of tartar.   The anasarca was by these means
relieved, but nothing more.   Even elaterium, which to all appearance totally
emptied her, left the urine unaltered.   Squill
rather irritated than unloaded.   Crystals of
tartar in large dilution somewhat kept down
the phlogistic habit, but at length brought
on a debilitating diarrhœa.   Tonics of all
kinds, even when the swellings were most
reduced, gave speedy marks of aggravating
every symptom.

She was scarified with some relief.   The
fluid discharged by this operation did not at
all coagulate by heat, very little by nitrous
acid, and left hardly any extract on evaporation.   The urine became for a few days
entirely devoid of serum.

Salivation was readily excited by mercurial frictions ; the debilitating effects of
this mineral soon followed, and the effusions
increased.

Digitalis gave so much relief, that I have
to lament it was not exhibited sooner.   It
produced a softness of her pulse, and diminished the swellings ; but some unconquer-

able obstruction to the circulation still remained; she continued to suffer severely from palpitations, nightly spasms, a pain in the region of the heart, and an inability of lying on the left side, though she could bear well the horizontal posture; and the urine but partially cleared.

The length of the complaint afforded us an ample opportunity of trying most of the popular and celebrated remedies, tincture of cantharides, blue vitriol, the alkaline salts with bitters, expressed juice of artichoke, broom-tea, &c. : the three first of these with bad effect, the others with none.

A sudden attack of convulsions, with violent head-ach, blindness, dilated pupil, and some degree of strabismus, which lasted several days, convinced me that fluid was accumulated on the brain; and she was twice relieved from this state, as rapidly as she had fallen into it.

An ascites at length came on; and for the few last months of her life she was tapped almost every week, in the whole fourteen times; a fluid being at the first, as well as at every subsequent operation, drawn off, resembling in appearance soap-water, not coagulating at all by boiling heat, very little by nitrous acid, but a good deal by the acetate of lead.   Flakes of lymph often obstructed the canula.

As the disorder advanced, she became bloated, and lost her colour and appetite; the urine was less loaded, and more putrescent; and she died in a state of the most complete emaciation.

This patient's illness continued for more than two years; and during the whole of that period, with the few exceptions before mentioned, she had discharged daily by the kidneys a considerable portion of the coagulable part of the blood. Such a loss, even if artificially produced, no one, I imagine, could bear for many months together, without its proper signs, a bloated and cachectic habit. I consider the pericardium to have been the membrane most affected, from the seat of the pain and her frequently preferring the horizontal posture; but some unlucky circumstance prevented my putting the truth of this conjecture to the test by dissection.

K

CASE III.

R. B. ætat. 40, very intemperate in the use of fermented liquors, and liable to severe fatigues at night, in the winter of 1809 became universally anasarcous; and his chest was affected very soon after. He attributed the attack to cold. He was treated by drastic purgatives and squills without the least good effect, but on the contrary an aggravation of all its symptoms. There was a very general anasarca; a suppressed cough; expectoration of bloody frothy sputa; pain under the right breast; difficulty of lying on that side; great dyspnœa; orthopnœa; frightful dreams; pulse 100, very obscure. The urine became turbid when cold, and deposited a copious, branny and lateritious, sediment. It coagulated at a very low heat, and in an unusual degree.

I directed venæ-section twice with considerable relief; and the blood, though rather watery appeared to be in an highly inflamed state, as buffy as is ever seen in a pleurisy. In addition to these, the application of a blister, and the use of half an

10

ounce of infusum digitalis three times a
day, with what mild laxatives the state of
the bowels demanded, speedily recovered
him ; and the urine became natural. His
pulse was for a day or two alarmingly
retarded.

In a few months, from some irregularity,
he had a slight relapse, and was again relieved by small doses of the fox-glove in
tincture, persisted in during some time.
Under this plan his health seemed pretty
well re-established. But his habits of life
led him into excess; and two winters after,
during the prevalence of very cold weather,
he was again seized with signs of inflammation upon his chest, and what I was alarmed
at more than any thing else, dark sanious
pleuritic sputa in the quantity of nearly
one pint a day. His urine was every way
loaded as before. This last symptom, as well
as the dyspnœa, was relieved by digitalis ;
but the bloody sputum gradually changed
into true fœtid pus, and in six weeks he
died tabid.

CASE IV.

E. J. ætat. 20, three months since, after unusual exposure to cold, became anasarcous, and complained of pain in her left side, with cough. She had been treated in vain with a variety of the common remedies, purges, squills, crystals of tartar, &c.

I found the urine serous and rather tinged with blood, skin bloated and pale, legs swelled, pulse 90, hard, abdomen flatulent; and she had a certain degree of dulness of apprehension, joined with deafness and tinnitus aurium. In the early part of her disorder, leeches had been applied to the head, on account of some pain there, which was never well defined.

Soon after she had been put under my care, she was attacked suddenly, and without any apparent cause, by a most violent vomiting and diarrhœa, with head-ach of the most excruciating kind, a sensation as if the scalp were lifted by an internal force, some indistinctness of vision, intolerance of light, &c. She continued many days in the most excessive agony, the pupils neither fixed nor at all dilated, and the understanding suffering now and then only a momentary eclipse. Some blood was drawn from the arm, and observed to be considerably inflamed; and a blister was applied, but without any relief. About twenty-four hours before death, she fell into an apoplectic stupor.

On examining the head, we found the veins of the pia mater turgid; in each of the lateral ventricles about half an ounce of blood loosely and recently coagulated, with some serum; the third and fourth ventricles filled with a similar substance: and the brain itself in the immediate neighbourhood of these last considerably injured in its texture. The hæmorrhage was traced to the basilary artery, which nearly at its bifurcation was dilated into an aneurismal sac of the size of a horse-bean, and appeared to have opened into the cavities of the brain at the communication between the third and fourth ventricles. A considerable quantity of pretty firmly coagulated blood was found under the membrane covering the tuberculum annulare and medulla oblongata; and this extravasation extended further down in the course of the medulla spinalis, than we could readily follow by dissection. ... The blood, though firmly coagulated, did not assume the form of successive layers, as is usual in aneurismal extravasations of any long continuance. The artery was entirely sound and natural in every other part of its course.

The lungs were sound. There were adhesions on both sides of the thorax, rather recent on the left; the fluid in the pericardium nearly natural. A few lymphy spots were observed on the heart.

The abdomen was free from any appearances of disease.

The cellular membrane of the whole body, and of the lower extremities particularly, besides containing a quantity of serous fluid, was loaded with a coagulated semi-transparent substance, similar to that described in page 110.

The very remarkable aneurism, which was the cause of death in this instance, was undoubtedly not the cause of the dropsy; nor can we reasonably consider it to have produced the inflammation of the blood; the anasarca itself therefore was of the inflammatory kind ; and in this dissection we have an opportunity, not often presented, of observing the effects of that disease, arrested, as it were, in the middle of its course.

CASE V.

M. B. ætat. 17, 1809, when she consulted me, had a considerable degree both of ana-sarca and ascites, a chorded pulse, dyspnœa, pain of the left side, with difficulty of lying on it, cough, urine scanty, lateritious, and greatly loaded with serum. I ventured to draw some blood, which was found buffy; and the operation gave great relief.

These symptoms had come on about six weeks before, on her recovery from a febrile attack, called typhus, but which had probably left some congestion, as on her beginning to take, by the advice of her officious neighbours, large doses of bark in substance for the improvement of her general health, the symptoms above related had rapidly made their appearance. The apothecary added, that squills had rather aggravated her complaints.

K 4

On scarifying the legs, much fluid was discharged from them, which gave hardly any signs of albumen by the common tests. The urine, at the same time, became copious and perfectly watery; so true is the remark of that excellent writer Van Swieten, that discharges from the legs often make a favourable change in the urine. *   But the effect seldom continues long; it soon ceased in this instance, and the danger of sloughs is certainly so great as to preclude their very general use.   Digitalis speedily and entirely relieved her.

CASE VI.

R. B. ætat. 35, accustomed to a sea-faring life, in which he had lately exposed himself much to rough weather, and been very intemperate, became in the course of ten days universally anasarcous, and felt some pain in his side, with cough and dyspnœa; the bowels costive, with tension of the abdo-

* Van Swieten Commentaria, 4to. tom. iv. p. 255.

men; the urine scanty, depositing a red sediment, and coagulating by heat.

Half an ounce of infusion of digitalis, twice a day, shortly recovered him.

CASE VII.

C. D. ætat. 40, was very extensively anasarcous, and somewhat oppressed in her breathing; bowels costive; urine natural in appearance, coagulating in some degree by heat. She attributed the attack, which was rather sudden, to checked perspiration.

She speedily recovered by the use of digitalis.

CASE VIII.

R. F. ætat. 40, very intemperate, and long subject to a pain of the right side, in the winter of 1809, after the most excessive use of strong liquors, and some exposure to cold, became rapidly anasarcous, and affected with cough and slight hæmoptoe. Bowels costive; urine coagulating.

Digitalis in very moderate doses soon carried off his bad symptoms. The next winter he had a similar attack, relieved by the same means; but he does not regain any robustness of health.

CASE IX.

E. D. ætat. 30, a corpulent woman, of a phlegmatic temperament, had swelled legs during her pregnancy. After her confinement, her symptoms increased rapidly to a true anasarca; and she had much cough. I found the urine to coagulate.

Digitalis entirely unloaded her; and she then took the Peruvian bark with great advantage.

These cases speak for themselves; and it is, I trust, unnecessary to recall to the reader's recollection those signs of inflammatory disposition, which occur in many of them; the cough, pain, and stricture of the chest in some, the hard pulse in others, the occasional inability of lying on the affected side, the buffiness of the blood, wherever it was drawn.   It is difficult to suppose, that the watery effusions are distinct from that character of inflammation, which we find so prevalent.   The principal danger arises undoubtedly from the latter, and from its great tendency to fix internally.   If it can be checked before the inflamed surfaces are much altered, there is hope : if this alteration has gone to any extent, there is none.

CHAPTER VII.

OF THE CACHEXY, WITH CASES AND A DISSECTION.

THE term, Cachexy, has not always been employed in the same sense by medical writers. Amongst the older physicians it was used to denote that remarkable state approaching to actual dropsy, in which the œdematous swellings are slight, but the depravation of the whole habit very considerable. Linnæus has most accurately and elegantly defined it by the words, *pallor corporis œdematosus cum debilitate et mœrore ;* and Boerhaave has entered very minutely into its history. We have on the other hand the great authorities of Cullen and Sauvages, who express by this term not one disease, but a whole class of diseases, including emaciation, swellings, and defœ dations of the skin. Dr. Cullen in particular, asserts, that what the ancients called cachexy, is the true dropsical habit, always the commencement of an universal dropsy, and therefore not requiring any separate consideration. It is certainly a dropsical habit, and disposed to terminate in the exquisite form of that disease, particularly if any attempt is made to remove it by inflaming and tonic remedies. But sometimes these patients, when the urine is greatly increased in quantity, as in the cases mentioned by Dr. Latham * and by Mr. Watts of Glasgow †, continue rather emaciated than truly dropsical; and Boerhaave has well stated amongst the confirmed symptoms of cachexy, *marcor vel leucophlegmatia et hydrops.* ‡ Van Swieten adds in his commentary, that if the urine is increased in quantity, the body wastes; if lessened, it swells. The latter is undoubtedly by far the most frequent occurrence. Altogether it differs so much from the common anasarca in its early symptoms, and often in its progress, that without any desire to restore obsolete

* Latham on Diabetes, p. 139.   † Watts on Diabetes, case iii. p. 74.   ‡ Boerhaave's Aphorisms, 1170.

terms, I think it necessary to give to the facts themselves a distinct consideration.

The cachexy is usually marked from the very first by some disorder of the abdomen. The patient is dispirited, has no appetite, and digests nothing. There is likewise, even before the swellings make any progress, a bloated, almost transparent, complexion, the truest proof of the body not being nourished. Where proper food is not abstracted, this deficiency can only have for its cause, either the imperfect conversion of food into chyle, or frequent losses of blood. Dr. Darwin describes the extreme of the former of these causes, when he asserts, that occasionally, the liver failing in its office of secretion, the body ceases to be nourished, and the complexion resembles the transparency of a full-grown silk-worm, with a yellow tint not greater than is natural to serum. He thinks these patients die from inanition and want of chyle, and even proposes tranfusion of blood. * A similar transparency of colour, though with more sallow-

* Darwin's Zoonomia, vol. i. sect. xxx. 1, 4. and vol. ii. 1, 2, 6.

ness, has been compared by Mr. John Bell to modelled wax, and observed by him to originate in small repeated discharges, as for example, the menorrhagia, the hæmorrhoidal flux, the bleeding from stumps after amputation, and even the leucorrhœa. He adds, that this complexion never quits the patient entirely, although he may recover from the disorder. In the present instance, both these causes seem to unite; the food is imperfectly assimilated, and the coagulable part of the blood, generally, at least, if not in every instance, passes off by the urine. At what period of the disease this discharge takes place, and what share it has in producing the other symptoms, is worthy of serious inquiry. I have seen it when the legs only just begin to swell; and lately in two cases of cachexy threatening an entire dropsy, it was to my surprize wholly wanting.

CASE I.

W. E. ætat. 70, of a gouty habit, and very intemperate mode of living, had been declining in health for nearly twelve months.

His skin was remarkably pale and transparent, the pulse nearly 100, low and intermitting, appetite very bad, bowels irregular, fæces pale, urine almost colourless.

He did not lie easily on the left side, and complained of a stricture about the lower part of the chest and hypochondria, with some wheezing, and expectoration of a few dark sanious sputa.

Suspecting a diseased liver, I ordered very mild mercurials, but without any good effect. He died not long after; a decided anasarca having at length come on, and the urine then examined being found serous. At what period this symptom began, it is now impossible to say.

CASE II.

W. N. ætat. 50, of intemperate habits; great feebleness and dejection of mind; complexion very pale and transparent; dyspnœa; short cough; stricture of the chest and hypochondria; loss of appetite; nausea ; looseness of the bowels ; fæces hardly coloured with bile ; legs slightly swelled ; urine pale, scanty, when cold uniformly turbid, and as white as if chalk had been mixed with it. It became clear on the application of heat, and then soon coagulated. After the use of a dose or two of calomel, it had been observed once or twice to deposit a bloody sediment.

These symptoms had been forming about six months, and he soon became more entirely dropsical.

Digitalis tried however cautiously, debilitated him ; squill acted not much better. Many mild diuretics were exhibited without effect. He pursued the same intemperate habits, and died not many months after.

CASE III.

E. B. ætat. 60, complexion pale and transparent ; ancles swelled ; pulse 80, weak and regular ; shortness of breathing ; cough ; indigestion ; irregular appetite, and occasional vomiting of a fluid that in smell

L

and taste she described as resembling Harrowgate water; fæces but little coloured; urine pale, natural in quantity, much loaded with serum.

These symptoms were of three months' duration; she had long suffered from the species of indigestion above described, and a fulness of the right side, for which she had been treated by several courses of mercury; but particularly the very free and continued use of crude quicksilver, advised by the late Dr. Warren. She soon became anasarcous, and was unable to lie down in bed. The œdema, as is common in scorbutic persons, frequently attacked and quitted a part almost instantaneously.

She could now hardly be prevailed on to try any remedies, and shortly afterwards died.

CASE IV.

Mary Bancroft, ætat. 58, Hospital, 1809. Her appearance was marked by great dejection and anxiety, and a very sallow bloated skin. I observed that the conjunctiva was not discoloured. There was considerable dyspnœa on motion ; the pulse 80, strong and quick ; slight swelling of the ancles ; a general fulness of the abdomen ; and many signs of a loaded stomach, with fœtid eructations and a bilious diarrhœa. Her urine was moderate in quantity, rather high-coloured, and coagulated by heat to a great degree.

Milder laxatives failing, I was tempted by the severe bilious symptoms to give a few doses of calomel, which somewhat relieved the bowels, but certainly debilitated much. A slight salivation followed, with increased dyspnœa and pain upon the chest; the urine became more loaded than usual, and then for the first time, as far as was observed, deposited a bloody mucous sediment. These circumstances induced me to draw off some blood which was highly inflamed. The operation gave great relief, and was afterwards repeated to the fourth time with similar advantage.

The tincture of digitalis was then directed in the quantity of seven or eight drops three times a day. It required as much laudanum to prevent its affecting the stomach and bowels, besides the frequent use of solid opium, and in that form was continued for more than two months, with a daily amendment of all her symptoms, and particularly of the state of the urine. At the end of that period she was reported cured.

About four months after, on exposure to cold, she was attacked with an inflammatory pain under the left breast, darting most acutely through the region of the heart to the blade-bone. It yielded to very large venæ-section and gentle purges. The urine was not again loaded. A lapse of more than three years has now confirmed her cure; and she is regaining a state of health and complexion much beyond what it was possible to calculate upon.

What share of her recovery is to be attributed to the opium, it is not easy to say. Dr. Mead cured by it one case of dropsy, which he supposed connected with preternatural heat and inflammation of the abdominal viscera, and quotes Dr. Willis's authority for some similar facts.* Dr. Heberden likewise speaks favourably of this remedy.†

* Mead's Monita et Precepta Medica, cap. 8th.
† Heberden's Commentaries, page 224.

CASE V.

R. B. ætat. 45; sallow and bloated skin; pulse 100, hard and redoubling; loss of voice; dyspnœa; inability of lying on the left side; stricture about the hypochondria; abdomen swelled, but giving no decided sense of fluctuation; frequent dark bilious discharges; œdema of the legs; eyes not tinged with bile; urine of the colour and appearance of rennet whey, copious at night, precipitating at 160°.

Six months before, she had been attacked with inflammatory pain of the right side, a large expectoration of bloody sanious sputa, called hepatic, and great disorder of the bowels. These symptoms had continued, though with less severity, ever since.

Soon after I visited her, there came on, from no apparent cause, a violent vomiting and constipation, attended by great oppression of the head. General convulsions succeeded, with a permanent stupor and fixed but not dilated pupil. The bowels at length yielded, and much black bile was dis-

charged, but in vain.   During this strug-
gle, which lasted four days, the œdema totally disappeared, the urine increasing in
quantity and passing off involuntarily.
Blood drawn on the third day was watery,
but much cupped.   Not more than two
hours before her death, the pulse remained
still quick and hard.

We found, on opening the head, inflammation of the pia mater; the vessels overloaded with blood; and about a table
spoonful of water in each of the lateral
ventricles.

In the thorax, the lungs were every where
free from adhesions, and bore no marks of
any inflammation extending from the liver;
but in the lower part of the right lung, there
were many small coagula of extravasated
blood, apparently seated in the cellular
membrane, from which source probably the
sanious sputa above mentioned originated.
About four ounces of bloody serum were
found on each side of the chest, and a small
quantity of pale fluid in the pericardium.

In the abdomen there was but little water;
the liver hard, with a thick curled edge, its
membrane being rather white and greatly

thickened, and the surface irregular with tubercles. A considerable portion of its substance was divided into hard brown tubercular masses; but this process was least marked in the central parts, and seemed to have begun superficially. The other viscera of the abdomen were sound; I speak particularly of the kidneys.

The absence of the bilious tinge in the eyes, and of the high colour of the urine, thought necessary signs of a scirrhous liver, is entitled to some notice; and I must request the reader particularly to attend to the state of the right lung, which I think demonstrates the origin of some of those spittings of blood connected with hepatic obstructions, without our having recourse to the supposition of an adhesion of parts, and an inflammation of the diaphragm itself.

The speedy termination of this case appears to have depended on a sudden dropsical metastasis to the brain, of which vomiting is a common sign.

The transparency of complexion above described is sometimes connected with a remarkable paleness or loss of colour, as in the three first cases. In these very little bile appeared to reach the intestines, and none certainly was absorbed. Dr. Darwin thinks that a torpor or palsy of the liver exists in such persons, and adds, that he has in vain attempted to stimulate them by calomel and steel. We cannot be surprised at this want of success, when we recollect that mercury, which corrects an inflamed or active liver, frequently adds to a feebleness of that gland; and patients fall into such a state, who have often undergone courses of mercury for its supposed or real obstructions. As to chalybeates, I have found them to be rapidly and uniformly injurious.

In cases IV. and V. there was a considerable sallowness, as well as transparency of skin, probably from excess of bile, since there certainly was an overflow of it into the intestines.

The presence of a bloody sediment in cases II. and IV., connected apparently with the use of mercury, is likewise entitled to some attention.

CHAPTER VIII.

CASES RESEMBLING LAND-SCURVY.

CASE I.

W. S. ætat. 40, 1800, of very temperate habits, was attacked about six weeks before I visited him, with febrile symptoms, attended by incessant vomiting of bile and constipation. He complained particularly of a pain and trembling in the region of the stomach, greatly increased by fermented liquors. After a few days this sensation was transferred from the stomach to the extremities, which became stiff and swelled, particularly at the ancles and knees. At the same time he was covered with petechiæ; and an affection of the wrists and shoulders took place, not wholly unlike that proceeding from the colic of lead.

In this state he consulted me.   I found his pulse 90, and rather hard, complexion sallow and very bloated, a pale purple colour of the lip, dejection, dyspnœa, and such a loss of strength that he could hardly walk about.   Round the ancles a slight impression of the finger was left on pressure ; but his joints generally, and particularly the bendings of the knees, were rather tense than œdematous.   There was some disposition to hæmorrhage from the nose.

The urine was amber coloured, moderate in quantity, and coagulable by heat. It was once or twice slightly tinged with blood.

It did not change the colour of infusion of litmus added to it within an hour after it was made*, and speedily putrefied.

His quitting the neighbourhood at this time prevented my attending to the case further.   My short experience of it showed

* I omitted to mention, that a similar experiment was tried in the case related in the Introduction, page v. with the same result.

me that he bore purging badly, and tonics still worse. I have since learnt that he became emaciated rather than dropsical, and died about twelve months after.

CASE II.

W. R. ætat. 50, of a very unhealthy habit, became suddenly feverish, and vomited bile, with great pain of the stomach and constipation ; about a week after, petechiæ appeared with some little relief, and as the termination of a febrile paroxysm.

This patient had, when young, been affected with sea-scurvy. For nearly two years he had declined in health and spirits, and suffered much from violent vertigo. Twelve months since, he had consulted me on account of what I then thought a threatening dropsy of the chest. Without examining the urine, I had directed calomel and squills, with one or two doses of which, as he informed me, he grew better. I saw him again about a month after the petechiæ had appeared, and found an irregular, intermittent, pulse, palpitations, dyspnœa, languor, loss of appetite, bilious vomiting and purging, sallow, bloated, complexion, conjunctiva yellow, the slightest possible œdema of the ancles, urine loaded with serum, but not high coloured ; which made me suspect that the yellowness of the eye was produced rather by an altered texture of the blood, than by bile.

The bark and vitriolic acid brought on a stricture of the chest ; neither did a free use of lemons and oranges, or of the antiscorbutic herbs, do any thing for him. He became dropsical, with signs of internal effusion, and died suddenly.

Blood drawn in the advanced stage of this complaint, for the relief of his breathing, was found to be very buffy.

CASE III.

W. H. ætat. 60 ; pale complexion ; anxiety ; weak pulse ; shortness of breathing ; legs œdematous, and covered with small pulpy tumours, which after inflaming, dispersed without bursting; a few petechiæ; urine scanty, made frequently and in small quantities, particularly at night; by heat, a little below boiling, it became very slightly clouded, and deposited an inconsiderable coagulum by nitrous acid. These complaints were of some weeks' duration.

The squill purged and nauseated him much, without any apparent advantage; but under the use of decoction of bark and diuretic salt he improved rapidly, and soon recovered his former health.

CASE IV.

W. R. ætat. 35, June, 1803, had been long in the habit of great excesses in diet, and a very free use of spirits. He had been subject to discharges of blood, considered hæmorrhoidal, to pains of the head, epistaxis, hæmoptoe, occasionally a nightly asthma, and what are called hypochondriac symptoms.

He had the influenza in 1803, and did

not well recover from it. His cough remained; and his legs began to swell. I perceived in him a considerable distress in breathing, and a sallowness of complexion, with a remarkable purple tinge of the lips. The urine was pale and coagulable. His dropsy increased. The legs at length began to discharge freely, and his breathing was so much relieved, that I ventured on the Peruvian bark. He thus became totally unloaded, and was thought to be recovering. But some inaccuracy of diet, of which he was frequently guilty, brought on a diarrhœa. To this, after it had continued not more than two days, succeeded a bloody salivation, and an eruption of petechiæ. A sphacelus appeared on the ulcerated spots on his legs, and he was shortly carried off. I could not learn that he had taken any mercurials which might possibly account for the salivation.

If the cachexy approaches to the land-scurvy by a similarity of symptoms, these four cases are brought still nearer to it by the addition of a petechial eruption. Two of them in particular can be hardly said to differ at all from the purpura minutely described by Dr. Willan.*

It is important to recollect that this disease is not characterized by sponginess and bleeding of the gums, as an essential symptom, that it originates in causes materially different from those which produce the sea-scurvy, and is apparently of a more inflammatory nature. In the two cases above alluded to, it was hardly possible to overlook the acuteness of the attack, the signs of inflammation in the upper part of the abdomen, and that remarkable metastasis to the surface of the body and the extremities. In some of these respects, they greatly resembled the case mentioned in the introduction to this work, as occurring at St. Bartholomew's Hospital, and in

* Willan on Cutaneous Diseases, vol. i. p. 467.

which nothing but the diabetic discharge of urine appears to have prevented * dropsy. Venæ-section would, I believe, have been their appropriate remedy; in the early stage, probably a successful one; nor does the presence of petechiæ furnish any insuperable obstacle to such an operation. Sydenham considered purple spots as the height of inflammation in fevers. Dr. Darwin † met with several examples of petechiæ, vibices, swelled legs and pulmonary hæmorrhage, which he calls scorbutic, attended by an inflamed blood; and Dr. Parry has inserted in the 5th volume of the Edinburgh Medical and Surgical Journal two instances of a similar nature. Such authorities stand in need of no addition, except in ascertaining the frequency of the occurrence.

An opinion of the great affinity between scurvy and dropsy has long prevailed; to which Sydenham alludes when he quotes the saying, *ubi scorbutus desinit ibi incipit*

* Introduction, p. v.
† Darwin's Zoonomia, vol. i. sect. xxvii. 2.

hydrops. * He considered it as the part of an erroneous doctrine then in fashion, by which almost all chronic diseases were at times pronounced scorbutic, and asserts the maxim to be true only in a more limited sense, that where the dropsy appears the preconceived notion with regard to a scurvy falls to the ground. But it seems to me not unaptly to delineate several of these cases, which are connected with dropsy by a resemblance in the urine, and by a general similarity of symptoms with the scurvy. Experience can alone show how far the coagulable state of this discharge extends in scorbutic cases. An assertion of Hoffman would lead us to believe that it is very common. He remarks, that in confirmed scurvy the urine is so loaded, that one pint of that fluid sometimes contains from three to four ounces of solid extractive matter, as ascertained by evaporation.†

In chronic petechiæ this symptom is

---

* Sydenham. Opera, p. 276. sect. vi. cap. v. de Rheumat.

† Hoffmanni Opera, tom. i. p. 379.

M.

certainly not always present. In some mild cases, in one very severe case distinguished by sponginess of the gums and hæmorrhages, in two where the legs were even swelled, no traces of it could be dis covered.

CHAPTER IX.

CASES OF HYDROTHORAX, IN WHICH THE URINE WAS COAGULABLE BY HEAT; WITH A DISSECTION, &c.

CASE I.

M. B. ætat. 40. Her legs were very slightly swelled; but the state of the urine, independent of other circumstances, would have instantly convinced me that these swellings were truly dropsical. It coagulated by heat much below the boiling. Her other symptoms were great debility and languor, with a sallow complexion, purple lips, abdomen greatly distended and tympanitic, pulse 120, weak, regular, inability of lying on either side, some orthopnœa, great dyspnœa, and harsh ineffectual

M 2

cough with much pain. She had been brought to bed about ten weeks before. During her pregnancy, she had suffered greatly from cough and pain of the right side. These increased much soon after her confinement, which she attributed partly to the cold lotions used at that period, for the purpose of stopping a severe uterine hæmorrhage.

She was, in so weak a state, that evacuations by purging could not be attempted. The fox-glove affected her violently in the smallest doses; and the preparations of squills seemed to increase her cough and difficulty of breathing. As she became oppressed with water, I thought it advisable to scarify the legs, which certainly was not done without temporary advantage; and whilst the discharge from them continued, the urine was more natural. She died soon after.

On examining the body, we found that the tympany observed during life was confined almost entirely to the stomach, which was excessively distended. There was some whey coloured fluid in the abdomen; the liver rather large, firm and pale, but not otherwise diseased; the kidneys remarkably small, and sound, if we except two or three hydatids of the size of a garden pea in the cortical part.

The right side of the thorax was completely overloaded with turbid water; the lung compressed to the size of a man's fist, and a very small quantity of pus, about half a tea-spoon full, deposited under the pleura pulmonalis, nearly as in the case described in page 95; the pleura costalis universally much inflamed, and covered with so thick a layer of lymph, as quite to obliterate its surface; on the left side, the lung sound, and its membrane free from any great mark of inflammation, whilst the pleura costalis on that side likewise was coated with lymph, and there was a great deal of serum in the cavity; pericardium containing rather an unusual quantity of fluid; heart natural.

CASE II.

J. R. ætat. 60, of a gouty habit; pulse 80, strong, full, intermittent; palpitations;

loaded countenance; cough; wheezing; dyspnœa much increased on motion; total inability of lying down in bed, till about two or three o'clock in the morning, when a little sleep is obtained, the suffocation in the beginning of the night being very dreadful; legs œdematous; hands slightly puffed; urine scanty, made frequently and with pain, and containing a branny sediment. Before it reached the boiling heat, it became slightly clouded, and deposited a few flakes.

Some years since he had been attacked by a palsy of the left side; the dyspnœa had been observed about six months; and the cough and nightly suffocation rather more than three.

Two drachms of infusum digitalis were ordered three times daily. Its diuretic effect followed rather unexpectedly in four or five doses, and was attended by a great relief of his symptoms. His life was undoubtedly prolonged some years by the cautious repetition of this medicine; and he at length died from complaints of a very complicated nature.

CASE III.

L. B. ætat. 30, was labouring under the most excessive dyspnœa, and orthopnœa, with an eager anxious countenance, very quick pulse, no sort of œdema, the urine pale, and coagulating at a low heat; complexion not sallow.

He had suffered for several springs a pain in the right side, relieved by gout in the extremities; but in the preceding month of March this pain never quitted the region of the liver, and was attended by a congestion of the abdomen, which had caused the exhibition of many mercurial laxatives. At present the fæces were rather thin, and totally devoid of bile. The dyspnœa had come on and increased very suddenly, being altogether not much more than of a week's duration.

The state of the urine, combined with other circumstances, made me attribute it to one of those rapid effusions on the chest which sometimes occur, although his complexion had none of that sallow paleness so common in this disease ; and I despaired of his recovery.

He took the digitalis with some relief for a few hours, but died two days after.

CASE IV.

J. R. ætat. 60, lame in the right leg in consequence of a scrophulous caries, was now labouring under decided marks of hydrothorax, for which he had been taking squills and calomel.

I found him in a salivation, suffering from the most excessive dyspnœa, the pulse hard, blood much cupped, urine pale and greatly loaded with serum.

Nothing could be done for him, and he died shortly after.

CASE V.

W. H. ætat. 48, pale and bloated, with a remarkable purpleness of the lips, but no œdema of the extremities; pulse 80, quick, irregular; fulness in the region of the stomach; flatulency; costiveness; great dyspnœa on motion; a harsh and dry cough; urine containing a red sediment, and coagulating by heat somewhat under the boiling.

He had been falling gradually into this state for nearly twelve months, and had been lately taking squill with some aggravation of his symptoms.

Fifteen drops of tincture of digitalis every eight hours gave considerable relief, and enabled him both to lie down in bed, and to walk up hill with ease. For these two last winters he has been obliged to return very cautiously to the same remedy, and always with advantage.

CASE VI.

R. C. ætat. 50, who had passed many years in the West Indies, and suffered from the disorders of that climate, consulted me by letter, from some distance, January

1808.   He described himself as sallow, and
rather bloated, but without any true œdema
even of the ancles ; as having an irregular
and intermittent pulse, a short cough, and
considerable dyspnœa after any exertion ;
awaking also from his first sleep in severe
suffocations and being unable to lie down
for the remainder of the night.   The
bowels were stated to be costive, and the
urine high-coloured and foul.   He added,
that he had tried calomel and squill by the
advice of a neighbouring practitioner without advantage, and squill alone in full
doses, with a great increase of debility and
loss of appetite.

I declined prescribing for him till the
state of the urine, with regard to heat, was
ascertained, and was soon after informed
by the attending practitioner, that on experiment it grew milky long before it boiled, when placed in a spoon over the candle.
From this circumstance, more than any
other, I recommended the digitalis, and
with sufficient confidence to make him
eagerly enter upon its use.   He took only
two drachms of the infusion, twice a day,
for a week.   His symptoms were wholly

carried off by it; but his pulse fell to 40; and for a day or two there was some alarm about him. A few weeks after he had strength enough to throw out gout.

Every winter since he has had a slight attack, though very careful about cold; and he takes at those times, by my advice, no more than ten drops of the saturated tincture of digitalis twice a day, which uniformly relieves him. A larger quantity than this affects the pulse unpleasantly. As he is a man of observation, I can trust to his report when he informs me, that on the attack, his urine is not only turbid, but grows milky by heat, and so continues till he takes digitalis, when it uniformly clears every way.

CASE VII.

W. L. ætat. 30, subject in his youth to scrophulous disease and a caries of the bones, had for many years past been resident in London. For the last twelve months he had suffered under symptoms considered at first asthmatic, but afterwards assuming the complete character of hydrothorax ; for which he was originally treated on the tonic plan with an increase of the dyspnœa ; soon after, by another physician with a salivation, that greatly debilitated him ; and from a third, with rather better effect, he took digitalis mixed with purgatives. He was at length recommended to try his native air.

When I was consulted for him in Exeter, I found him very weak and emaciated, with an irregular pulse never less than 120 in the minute, anasarca, cough, sputa slightly tinged with blood, pain of the right side of the thorax, and spasms extending down the whole of that arm. Mixed with these, there was a great deal of load in the abdomen, and other symptoms resembling the spasmodic asthma. The urine was generally pale and not otherwise remarkable ; but when the dyspnœa was most severe, it grew foul and lateritious, and slightly coagulated under the boiling heat.

This is one of the few instances which I have met with where such a character was temporary; perhaps it may occur in asthmatic cases more than in any other.

Purgatives partially unloaded and relieved him; digitalis rendered very little, if any, service; and he died suffocated.

I learnt that the smallest dose of mercury had always injured him; and squill had usually augmented the dyspnœa to a most distressing degree.

There was some obscurity in this case, which could have been cleared up by dissection only. The evidence of water in the chest was considerable; but there seemed still greater reason to believe that the viscera themselves were unsound.

CASE VIII.

J. T. ætat. 30, January, 1812, was recommended from London to this neighbourhood for the sake of the climate. I found his expectoration beyond any doubt purulent, his legs swelled, abdomen somewhat bloated, breath short with complete orthopnœa, urine scanty and high-coloured, depositing much sediment, and coagulating in some degree by heat.

In other respects there was a certain firmness of habit, which made me think him capable of bearing squills. He was not cachectic in his colour, was desirous of food, and appeared to digest it.

I directed for him forty-five drops of the vinegar of squill every six hours. In the course of two days he was enabled to lie horizontally in bed; the swellings disappeared, and his urine entirely cleared in colour, sediment, and coagulum.

I consider it possible that, with such stamina, the ulcer of the lungs may yet heal.

CASE IX.

R. N. ætat. 60, subject to irregular gout and dyspepsia. I found his pulse quick, skin hot, considerable dyspnœa on motion and even on speaking, great orthopnœa, nightly suffocations, an inability of lying on either side, a very anxious countenance, legs œdematous and spotted with a few petechiæ, the urine rather copious, pale, crude, without any sediment, but coagulating at a low heat. There were likewise much indigestion and vomiting.

These symptoms had been gradually forming for many months. They indicated unequivocally an exudation into some cavity of the thorax; and a remarkable load about the heart, with a sense of fluctuation there often complained of by himself, convinced me that the pericardium was the membrane most affected.

Squills had been tried without any advantage. The digitalis was then directed. It was exhibited in the quantity of half an ounce of the infusion daily, and certainly showed very considerable power over the disease, by palliating the most urgent symptoms, and rendering the urine in every respect more natural. He was enabled to throw out a slight gout.

As however the complaint was by no means carried off, the remedy was continued in smaller quantities. During the use of no more than two drachms of the infusion daily, a pain came on over one of his eyes. He complained of great disturbance of his brain, which he himself referred to the draughts ; and within twenty-four hours this symptom was followed by a watery exhausting diarrhœa and low delirium. General convulsions speedily ensued, in which there was complete insensibility and foaming at the mouth, with an almost total cessation of the action of the heart. From this state he was recovered by an opiate injection.

Similar paroxysms returned two or three times during the next three weeks. In the intervals he became forgetful, delirious, and felt much pain in the head.

The anasarca totally disappeared, discovering the most excessive emaciation ; his posture in bed became nearly natural, but his urine still coagulated ; and in one of these convulsions he expired.

———————

Case I. is an example of hydrothorax connected with a very inflamed state of the membranes, and also of the lung. The deposit of pus under the pleura pulmonalis exactly resembled that mentioned in the article scarlatina. * We see how perfectly impossible recovery was in the advanced stage, and how very different a system from that of diuretics was proper at any period. Perhaps there was a time when a paracentesis might have rendered service.

In many instances it is probable that the internal membranes continue for a long period but little defaced, and still capable of some absorption ; in consequence of which, relief is obtained by small doses of medicine for many years together ; but the parts seldom recover their proper tone, and are disordered by every irregularity, but particularly intemperance and cold.

Dissections are wanting to explain their exact state.

The prevalence of this disease in the gouty habit, and the relief which gout driven to the extremities gives, persuade me that the slow and insidious process here suspected is often of that nature.

I likewise observe, that relief is more common, when there is a sediment, even of a pink colour, in the urine, than when there

* Page 95.

N

is none.   It indicates indeed fever, but some strength of constitution to throw it off. .

There is a cough to which old gouty habits are liable in the winter-season, with milder symptoms than those described in the preceding part of this chapter, and yet sufficiently severe to excite great alarm and distress.   The following is an example of it.

E. L. ætat. 63, of a florid complexion, liable to yearly fits of gout, and whose nephew forms the subject of one of the preceding cases, in the winter of 1807 did not throw out this disorder to the extremities, but had a violent harsh cough, with nightly restlessness and fever, swelled legs, and some degree of dyspnœa.   Squills relieved him.   The next year he fell into the same state, and that remedy entirely failed.   On examining the urine, which his complexion and general appearance had not hitherto induced me to suspect, I found it to coagulate by heat, and to be rather high-coloured, though without sediment.

Change of air and the return of warm weather for that time relieved him.   He ceased to reside in this county, and died the next winter.

I have known digitalis greatly disagree with these coughs; but whether from inaccuracy of dose, or the entire impropriety of the remedy, I cannot yet determine.

The reader may perhaps be of opinion, that case III. is of this kind, rather an example of gouty suffocation than hydrothorax.

CHAPTER X.

CASES OF ASCITES, IN WHICH THE URINE WAS COAGULABLE BY HEAT, WITH A DISSECTION, AND REMARKS.

CASE I.

R. H. ætat. 60, pale and bloated; ascites; no anasarca; urine slightly opaque under the boiling heat.

A pain of the right side, with dyspepsia, and his very intemperate habits induced suspicions of a diseased liver; but he sunk rapidly under a mercurial course.

CASE II.

L. M. ætat. 13, suffered from a severe peritonitis, at the same time that I was at-

14

tending, in consultation with Dr. Parr, her mother who died of the puerperal form of that disease. The daughter survived; but her abdomen became distended and fluctuating. The urine, clear and without sediment, grew milky under the boiling heat. There was not the least anasarca.

The navel soon after burst; and there were discharged from two to three quarts of sero-purulent fluid, with a complete subsidence of the swelling.

She changed the air and gained strength; and I learn that, after the fluid had collected and discharged a third time, the orifice quite healed, and she perfectly recovered.

CASE III.

R. Forward, ætat. 32, very intemperate in the use of fermented liquors, was infected with syphilis some years since by her husband, and had undergone repeated irregular salivations with partial relief. She was admitted into the hospital as an in-patient, for the remains of that complaint, but soon afterwards, at her own desire, went into the country, where for more than six months she kept herself under a constant course of mercurial friction, both whilst pregnant and after her delivery. She was re-admitted under my care, 1810, on account of the debility which this course had occasioned.

There was a very considerable ascites, with some slight swelling of the lower extremities, a total loss of appetite, glossy red tongue, irritable bowels, and a low pulse. The urine, far from being scanty, was made in the quantity of two quarts every night, and about one quart in the day. It was pale, without the least sediment, and coagulated by heat.

Sarsaparilla passed through the bowels rapidly. By the exhibition of two or three small doses of digitalis, the ascites was somewhat relieved, but only to give way to tympany; and such debility and diarrhœa ensued, as made it necessary to support her by wine and cordials. From this situation she rallied, could not bear the smallest dose of digitalis, and fell at length into a completely typhoid state, with brown crust of the tongue, repeated aphthæ, sordes about the teeth, refusal of all food, and a gradual reduction of the swellings. The bark at all periods produced an increased and painful tension. She died after lingering in this state more than six weeks.

On examining the body, we found that the puffy node on the forehead concealed a caries which reached to the frontal sinus. In the body of the tibia likewise was a large abscess.

On the right side of the abdomen a considerable visceral hardness was felt externally. It was produced by the remarkable shape and enlargement of the right lobe of the liver. The whole of that gland was unusually weighty and solid, with membranous thready marks on its surface, when cut, firmly resisting the knife, and of a texture resembling the incipient scirrhus. Its edges were blunt, rounded, and thick; and its size unusually great. A natural variety perhaps contributed to this bulk; for whilst the right lobe projected downwards in a thick large mass, the left was subdivided into several lobules, so as to expose almost the whole of the gall-bladder. The concave surface of the liver was somewhat connected to the neighbouring parts by membranous adhesions, as was likewise the spleen. The gall-bladder was filled with a dark green bile. The other viscera were sound, except the kidneys, which were remarkably solid and hard, and their structure somewhat confused. I considered it approaching to scirrhus. In the cavity of the abdomen there was about a pint of serum, which coagulated by heat more firmly than usual. The heart was very small ; the lungs sound, adhering to the pleura in some places, and their cavities containing no fluid.

———

The purulent fluid discharged from the cavity of the abdomen in case II. is worthy of particular notice, especially as there was not the least appearance of any other dropsical accumulation which might be thought to supply, by absorption, the serum present in the urine.

I request the reader to connect case III. with those related chapter VI. section II. under the article, mercury. The hardness and enlargement of the liver probably originated in the excessive use of spirituous liquors; but it is at least worthy of remark, that the freest and most continued exhibition of mercury afforded no relief; how far it aggravated the complaint is a more doubtful question.

There is something likewise very uncommon in the state of the kidneys here described. *   I am not aware that such a hardness approaching to scirrhus has ever been attributed to the use of mercury; yet in another case, where mercury had been employed to a great extent, the kidneys were observed to be unusually firm †

* See Baillie's Morbid Anatomy, p. 181. (article, Kidney Scirrhous.)
† Page 109.

CHAPTER XI.

CASES OF HYDROCEPHALUS, IN WHICH THE URINE WAS COAGULABLE BY HEAT, OR CONTAINED A BLOODY SEDIMENT ; WITH A DISSECTION, &c.

THE following cases of hydrocephalus internus might perhaps with equal or more propriety have been arranged under the several heads of scarlatinous and mercurial dropsy; but the accumulation to which they relate is of so much importance, that I prefer placing them in a separate article.

CASE I.

J. W. ætat. 10, excruciating pain in the forehead, attended by the most incessant screams; squinting of the left eye; pupil fixed, but not dilated; frequent and violent convulsions of the whole body; pulse 60, irregular in strength and number, and often intermitting; urine foul, dark-coloured, depositing, as soon as it was made, a sediment slightly tinged with blood, and giving a large coagulum at a very low heat. No part of the body was œdematous. The bowels had been regularly opened.

I entertained no doubt, that this was a case of incipient hydrocephalus; and indeed, whoever candidly reads the whole of this statement, must be of the same opinion, unless he has commenced his studies on these subjects with determining, that water in the head is never cured.

This child had suffered about a month before from scarlatina, the symptoms of which had not been very severe; a fortnight afterwards he had become anasarcous, and appeared to be relieved by a few purgatives, united with squills; the anasarca, however, had left him in a sudden manner, and from that time h. had complained of pains in his head, which rendered him heavy and ill-disposed to move.   On the morning of that evening on which I saw him, he had waked after a disturbed night, totally blind, and with the symptoms before detailed.

Not willing to wait for the slow operation of leeches, I requested that the temporal artery might be opened, which was done with great adroitness, ten ounces of blood being drawn off very rapidly.   The head was somewhat relieved by this operation. . His bowels were then unloaded by a colocynth injection, and a dose of jalap, to which was added a quarter of a grain of digitalis.   A large cap-blister was likewise applied, covering the whole scalp, and three drachms of infusion of digitalis given every eight hours.   Under this plan the convulsion speedily ceased ; correct vision returned ; and the urine became natural.

A few days after, whilst this remedy was still continued, some pain of the head returned, with great confusion of thought, and the urine was again observed to be tinged with blood.   It likewise precipitated by heat, but not till it began to boil ; and the coagulum was so loose, that I was very confident, from former observation of this fact *, tonics were demanded. He accordingly took the cinchona in substance, and speedily recovered. Three years have now confirmed his cure.

CASE II.

J. E. ætat. 7, of a scrophulous habit, and whose father had died phthisical some years before, was affected, June, 1804, with common febrile symptoms attended by vomiting and costiveness. For the purpose of opening the bowels, repeated doses of calomel were given at very short intervals, and the object fully obtained in the discharge of black liquid stools, such as are not only brought off by mercury but often entirely caused by it. To produce this result, two scruples of calomel had been given in forty-eight hours.

I was consulted on account of a very sudden prostration of strength, that followed. It was attended with a soreness of the gums, some effort at salivation checked by

* Pages 88 and 89.

an exhausting diarrhœa in which the stools were devoid of bile, a pulse irregular in number, strabismus, and low delirium. These increased in a few days to stupor, hemiplegia, convulsions, &c. which shortly terminated the scene. The urine was likewise observed to be very foul and greatly loaded with a most offensive bloody sediment, no blister having been at that time applied.

On examining the head, we found the veins of the pia mater turgid, that membrane inflamed, the lateral ventricles distended and containing nearly three ounces of watery fluid, which was more turbid than usual and coagulated both by heat and acids in a degree not common. The surface of the ventricles appeared dull and clouded, the neighbouring brain very soft and covered with red points.

I more particularly noticed the condition of the surface of the ventricles, because it is undoubtedly membranous, and proved indeed by anatomical demonstration to be a direct continuation of the arachnoid coat. In respect to their covering, therefore, they resemble other perfect cavities, and we may reasonably suppose them to be liable to the same processes both of health and disease; amongst the latter of which, an inflammatory dropsical effusion is perhaps the principal.

———

Case I. we must acknowledge to have been, in its termination at least, very unusual; but I hope, that the treatment so successful in it may be advantageously followed.

Dropsical metastases, particularly from the chest to the head and the contrary, have been often mentioned by practical authors; this is an example of metastasis from the extremities to the head, and favours an opinion, that such accumulations are rather of an active than a passive kind.

Case II. which I beg the reader to compare with case III. page 34, is, I fear, one only amongst many instances, in which calomel, pushed to an improper extent in very young persons, has been productive of the most fatal results. A general opinion prevails, that their constitutions resist mercury in a remarkable degree. Its entrance into the system they certainly do resist, more than we could expect; but they are greatly overcome by salivations; and the possible occurrence of such accidents may well set us constantly on our guard.

These few cases furnish no decided inference with regard to the state of the urine in hydrocephalus generally. An hydropic habit is probably attended by its proper constitutional signs, on whatever part it falls; but when scrophula or other causes locally affect the brain and produce an effusion, we are by no means entitled to expect the same changes in the blood and the secretions, as are observed in original dropsies. But experiment should in future supersede all conjectures on this subject.

CHAPTER XII.

RECAPITULATION.

FROM the foregoing cases it is evident, that the urine of dropsy assumes very different, and even opposite, appearances; and that though it often errs, as indeed we might expect it always would, by an excess of colour, sediment, and extractive matter; yet that sometimes it verges towards the opposite extreme, is apparently little animalized and crude, does not seem to possess the appropriate characters of urine, and is, I suppose, particularly deficient in what the chemists have lately called urea. I consider the former of these to indicate a strength of constitution, but an internal obstruction, and to require both active diu-

o

retics and deobstruents*; the latter to denote a feeble and impoverished habit, either
simply, or combined with great disease and
with an entirely broken state of health.†

In the midst of these extremes it need
not surprize us that, if the constitution is
not greatly shocked, or the extravasation
be small, this secretion should occasionally
differ but little from the healthy state. ‡

In addition to those characters which are
discoverable by mere inspection, there is
another infinitely more important, its property of coagulation by heat. §   This property is not connected exclusively with any
particular situation of the accumulated
fluid, nor with the affection of any particular organ.   It very generally, although
not uniformly, attends what may be called
original dropsy, and frequently is superadded to great visceral unsoundness; and
there cannot be a more fruitful source of
error in practice, than to consider it as an
evidence of mere debility, a term so incor-
rectly applied to several different species of

* Chapter IV.   † Chapter II.
‡ Chapter III.   § Chapter V.

disordered action. In short, it occurs under a great variety of circumstances, and
where, from a resemblance of other symptoms, it has been most expected, is sometimes absent. The laws that regulate its
appearance, what it denotes, and what it
requires, have been hitherto almost equally
unnoticed.

But is it possible, that such facts can be
indifferent? or, will any one flatter himself
that he understands an individual dropsical
case, whilst he overlooks this important
feature of it? The neglect, which it has received from practitioners in general, makes
me almost mistrust myself, when I estimate
it so highly; and I should be unwilling to
strain any consideration in medicine, as is
too often done, beyond its reasonable and
proper value. But it really does appear to
me, that a more correct application of diuretic remedies is one only amongst the many
advantages which may be derived from this
distinction; and that it will hereafter be
found capable of explaining many doubts,
of reconciling many apparent anomalies,
and of affording an insight hitherto rather
desired than expected into the state of the

blood and the secretions.   I shall therefore
dedicate the remaining pages to a more
complete investigation of its nature, founded in a great measure on the preceding
cases, partly on others which it is unnecessary to detail.

Of the encysted dropsies I have design-
edly omitted to speak ; because, as the
very term implies, consisting of accumulations not diffused through the natural cavities, but confined to cysts usually either
hydatids or an enlarged viscus, they admit
neither of the same explanation nor the
same relief that is applied to the disorders
of serous membranes.

The ovarian dropsy, the most common
of these, can be viewed only in the light of
an enlarged viscus ; and I have not found
the urine to be distinguished by any very
remarkable qualities.

CHAPTER XIII.

OBSERVATIONS ON DROPSIES WITH COAGULABLE URINE, DERIVED FROM THE PRECEDING CASES, &c.

IN treating of dropsies distinguished by a coagulable state of the urine, it appears to me desirable to bring first into view those facts, which relate to the nature and degree of that coagulation, and whatever else there may be remarkable in the urinary discharge.

In the succeeding sections of this chapter the symptoms of the disease are described, both where the dropsy is universal, and where it is confined to a single cavity. As the effects however of water pressing on any particular organ must be nearly the same, whatever be its constitutional cause,

o 3

little novelty can be expected in this detail. Nor indeed could I flatter myself that the history of the general symptoms would be agreeable to nature, if it did not in most important respects coincide with the descriptions of dropsy given by preceding writers. I have found it however necessary so far to deviate from the common arrangement, as to include in my description some cases of Cachexy distinguished rather by emaciation than swelling. The character of the urine has proved these to be of a truly dropsical nature; and nothing but an increased quantity of that discharge, however bad its quality, has prevented the appearance of anasarca. In some of them the increase is so great as to constitute a diabetes; and I have thought these entitled to particular notice in the last section of this chapter, under the name of *Diabetes Serosus.*

The remaining chapters are occupied with the causes and treatment of the disease.

SECTION I.

General Appearances of the Urine.

THE coagulation which takes place in dropsical urine is very various in its extent. Sometimes this fluid becomes opaque and milky at 160° or less, and soon breaks into small coagula, or even forms further into a mass nearly solid. *   In other instances it undergoes no alteration till it almost arrives at the boiling heat, becomes then slightly opaque but not milky, and gives a precipitate both small in quantity and loose in its texture.   More rarely, although the change is inconsiderable before it boils, the least evaporation converts it into a tremulous mass. †

The exact state of dilution, in which the serum is present, is not very easy to be de-

---

* Page 125 ; and Rollo on Diabetes, p. 447 and 448.
† Page 101.

o 4

termined.   Undiluted serum coagulates in
a mass, into the composition of which it is
evident that much water enters ; whilst the
coagulated part of this secretion is more
separated from its water, more opaque, and
resembling lymph or curd ; and I have not
been able by any artificial dilution of serum
to produce exactly the same appearances
of coagulation.   In one case and that not
apparently the most severe, I obtained from
four ounces forty grains of a firm white
coagulum, which lost by moderate desiccation one-fourth part of its weight, and
was in the proportion of two ounces to the
quantity of urine discharged daily. *   In
another, there remained on the strainer
seventy-five grains from four ounces, in the
proportion of ten drachms daily, which was
softer and was reduced by moderate desiccation to nearly one-half of its † weight.
In its least degree it barely tinges the boiling fluid. ‡

The nitrous acid produces a similar
effect ; and perhaps may sometimes suc-

* Page 105.   † Page 126.   ‡ Pages 166, 172, 180.

ceed, where the application of heat fails. But the latter of these shows both the extent and mode of coagulation with much nicer precision : and besides the superior facility with which it is employed, it has the great advantage of leaving the fluid free for further experiment.

The oxymuriate of mercury, which detects very minute quantities of albumen, is a test not particularly useful here ; since it acts on the urine in many other cases of dropsy *, and in some inflammatory disorders ; nor is it yet ascertained, to what extent this coagulum consists of albumen.

Infusion of galls produces a large precipitate ; the fluid strained after coagulation by heat, is of course less affected by this test, and has been found to leave but a small extract on evaporation.

This kind of urine is not unfrequently tinged with red blood †, and occasionally deposits pieces of lymph, and a bloody and very offensive sediment which does not redissolve by heat. ‡

* Page 64.   † Pages 132, 145, 154.
‡ Pages 88 to 93, 147.

In other respects it varies much, and in nothing more than in quantity, being sometimes very copious, so as almost to assume the character of diabetes *, more frequently scanty. It is rarely high-coloured, when made, but often deposits a branny and lateritious sediment, or even a white one, as if chalk had been mixed with it †, rarely of a bright pink colour; it likewise putrefies soon, and at least within an hour after it has been made, has been found to have no effect on vegetable blues. ‡

In some cases, on the other hand, it appears remarkably devoid of those sensible properties which commonly distinguish urine, and is probably deficient in urea. In this state it is perfectly clear and aqueous, apparently unanimalized, and what has been called crude; shows an excess of acid by reddening infusion of litmus, which property it long retains, and continues for a much longer period free from any evident

* Introduction, page iv.; pages 104 and 182; and Watts on Diabetes, page 74.

† Page 145. ‡ Page 154, and note in that page.

decomposition. * It at length putrefies. The quantity of animal matter which it contains would lead us always to expect a very rapid putrefaction; and there must be something extraordinary in its other combinations, which enables it in any instance so long to resist that process. It would be of great practical importance to pursue this inquiry further, and likewise to determine on the other hand by accurate experiments, whether the serous urine, at the time of its being made, is ever without an excess of acid; and still further, whether it is in any degree actually alkaline. I have occasionally tried some other common re-agents, such as the acetate of lead, pure ammonia, muriate of barytes, &c. but without any very important or satisfactory results.

This discharge has seldom been observed without some signs of dropsy, although they may be as yet apparently slight, amounting to nothing more than an œdema of one leg †, or a generally bloated habit. ‡

---

* Pages 105 and 126. † Introduction, page v.
‡ Pages 154 and 156.

At what precise stage of the disease it begins, whether gradually or at once, and whether it ever precedes the dropsical symptoms, would be a task of some labour to ascertain ; certainly, when it has once formed, it continues with a very considerable regularity, most severe perhaps before there is much anasarca, and gradually rather declining towards the fatal termination ; though even this uniformity of its continuance I do not consider to be a constant law. *

With the first appearances of amendment, the urine becomes more diluted. This favourable change particularly follows scarifications † and tapping ; but it then generally lasts only a few days.

The blood, in most instances in which it has been drawn, has been found buffy, often much cupped ‡, and remarkable even as it escapes from the vein, watery and of a dull colour very opposite to florid. The quan-

* Page 172.   † Page 136.
‡ P. 100, 103, 106, 123, 130, 133, 135, 147, 150, 156. Watts on Diabetes, p. 83.

tity and firmness of the albumen in the urine bear usually a direct proportion to the appearances of inflammation. Some portion of it, however, is consistent with a condition very opposite to the inflammatory, and even where Peruvian bark has effected a cure. * With regard to the absence of inflammation, much may be determined by the looseness of the coagulum, and the high degree of heat required for its precipitation. Thus distinguished, I have known it re-appear with signs of great feebleness in the constitution, where digitalis has been continued too long, and after all the accumulations have been† removed. Similar effects have speedily followed the use of mercury given improperly, and during the existence of an internal ulcer. ‡

* Page 123.   † Page 89.
‡ Pages 113, 114, 115.

SECTION II.

Symptoms of Anasarca and general Dropsy, including Cachexy, &c.

The diffused and general dropsy here described sometimes come on very suddenly and in habits previously sound; often their approach is more gradual, being apparently the result of, what is called, a broken state of health.

The dropsy which takes place after scarlatina is of the former kind; and if it be considered of much importance to trace the discharge from its commencement, will afford us the most favourable means of doing so. It is likewise observed particularly in those cases where the intensity of inflammation has fallen rather on the skin than the throat, after a mild disease, hardly ever in consequence of the severer form of it, the angina maligna; and I have thought, that a discreet use of the cold affusion has prevented its occurrence.

From a very obvious difference in the character of the swellings, it has been divided into the hot and cold œdema. The former comes on from a week to ten days after the disappearance of the eruption, and is attended by a fresh accession of fever, with great restlessness and irritation. The joints speedily become painful and swelled, particularly the knees, ancles, and wrists, and in a form greatly resembling the acute rheumatism, or rather gout; I have even noticed an extravasation of fluid in the large bursa above the knee ; and the pains to dart in the course of the muscles. In a few days more the swellings gradually subside, or change into a true œdema.

Not unusually the anasarca shows itself without much pain or inflammation, and the face and extremities become suddenly bloated. This takes place with a less exact limitation as to time than the former, even as late as a month after the decline of the efflorescence, and when the patient has been apparently recovering his strength. I speak with greater precision to the coagulable state of the urine in the latter case, than in the former.

A dropsy of the large cavities very commonly ensues ; in this way the abdomen is often affected ; but the thorax is more disposed to show signs of inflammation. As however the viscera are for the most part sound, it is commonly the fault of the practitioner if any fatal mischief takes place. From this probability of recovery I must except the hydrocephalus, in which the parts concerned are of so tender a structure, as seldom to bear much pressure without irreparable injury to their organization.

The urine in this attack is often singular even in its appearance, being turbid when made, of a very offensive smell, and resembling water in which flesh had been washed, as has been already remarked by Burserius. On standing it becomes clear, and deposits a bloody sediment. I have suspected that this state sometimes followed the very free use of calomel, a practice much too indiscriminately resorted to in the febrile complaints of children ; but I cannot deny that it has appeared, where not only no mercury, but no medicine of any other kind, had been exhibited during the whole ill-

I I

ness. * It should, however, give an immediate alarm. It is the effect of an aggravated hydropic habit, and requires the utmost activity as well as caution on the part of the practitioner.

In young and scrophulous subjects, this tendency to effusion, is apt to be speedily translated to the brain; and sometimes with a most terrible violence. A pain between the brows and heaviness of a few days' duration are succeeded by symptoms of hydrocephalus that cannot be misinterpreted; a pulse preternaturally slow and irregular; convulsions; inability to bear the upright posture; frequent exclamations of Oh! my head! the most incessant screams, as if the skin were pinched; blindness; strabismus; dilated pupil; and in the very last stage again, a great rapidity of circulation, with paralysis on one side of the body, whilst the other is convulsed.

The emaciation, in such instances, is observed to be singularly rapid; what is commonly the effect of an atrophy of many months, taking place in a few days.

* Page 92.

P

A slow and interrupted pulse is likewise amongst the most distinctive symptoms of incipient pressure on the origin of the nerves ; and hardly ever, I believe, originates in children from any other cause. Its presence is nearly conclusive.

The * anasarca generally disappears in a very delusive manner at the beginning of this attack on the brain, as if connected with the translation of some inflammatory process ; for that a mere feebleness and loss of tone should suddenly be transferred to a distant part, carries with it no air of probability. A similar metastasis has been observed from the chest to the head. Both in adults and children, convulsions often give the first warning of this sudden change of the seat of the disorder †, whilst in the primary and original hydrocephalus many other decided symptoms precede this.

The dropsy from drinking cold water is likewise acute, and speedily follows the

* Page 187.   † Page 128

application of the exciting cause. The same suddenness of attack is sometimes observable, where the cause is less obvious, but usually in the opinion of the patient connected with the external application of cold. Obscure chilliness is succeeded by heat and increased action, such as the phlegmatic constitutions most liable to these complaints are capable of raising, and particularly by a pain in the side. But the attention is soon diverted from these to the anasarcous swellings, which come on to a greater extent, and with more rapidity than are observed in any other instances. I have known a single fortnight completely sufficient for this effect; and the vulgar have attributed it to witchcraft. An œdema is now and then propagated over the whole body from one of the lower extremities, which for a few days had been observed to be rather painful and tense. * The scarlatina likewise furnishes examples of this kind †; and Dr.

* Pages 126 and 126.   † Page 87.

p 2

Monro mentions a similar fact in consequence of a sprain of the wrist. *

The mechanical pressure of these diffused
swellings will of course affect the breathing
to a considerable degree; but the harsh
cough, discoloured sputa, stitches in some
part of the thorax, and inability of lying
on one side, show that the cause of this
dyspnœa is often more deeply seated. The
abdomen likewise becomes bloated, with
thirst, costiveness, and some difficulty of
procuring discharges. The pulse is generally
hard or obstructed, and rising on blood-
letting; the blood inflamed.

This disease, if treated with indiscriminate remedies, proceeds to a fatal termination. The patient falls gradually into a
cachectic state, and loses his appetite and
digestion. Water accumulates in most of
the great cavities; least frequently perhaps, when the patient is of mature age, in
the ventricles of the brain, but very suddenly; and the absorption from that part
has been known to be as sudden as the de-

* Monro on Dropsy, page 10.   Note.

position. * In the thorax, it is most common, most distressing, and productive of the greatest anxiety of mind. In some instances a sudden death happens from this cause, in others a more lingering one, connected with sloughing ulcers of the lower extremities.

In the last stage, the dropsy often disappears; the abdomen becomes flaccid; and a superficial observer might think some great relief were at hand. But the urine is never natural; a tympany succeeds to the ascites; the strength and nervous influence daily fail; the brain appears affected; and the scene is not closed, till after the most complete emaciation has taken place. Nor do I know any sign more delusive, than a subsidence of the swellings, and an increased quantity of urine, if the character of it be not improved.

The natural cure is effected, either by a copious flow of diluted urine, which, if not strictly speaking spontaneous, is at least unexpected, and originates in circumstances of diet thought trifling, or by

* Page 128.

p 3

excessive discharges from the legs. A diarrhœa and sweating very rarely supply the place of these.

It is not to be supposed that the sudden and universal anasarca, here described as particularly following scarlatina and the extraordinary action of cold, is the most common form of the disease. Often the exciting cause, particularly if connected with intemperance, operates less immediately and by repeated impressions; in consequence of which the accumulations are more gradual and apparently milder in their symptoms, but with much greater difficulty carried off; their prevalent character, however, appears to be the same, and will certainly be best illustrated by contemplating attentively the more marked and unmixed cases.

A purulent expectoration * is not very unusual, either as the result of that same distemper of the constitution which

* Pages 131, 173.

produces the dropsy and in such instances has affected more than one order
of parts, or as preceding it, and predisposing to it, and materially altering its
nature.

Sometimes the principal severity of
the disorder falls; from the very first, on
the viscera of the abdomen. The patient
has been sallow, and not positively well
for some weeks; and at length, in consequence of some occasional cause not
always correctly ascertained but referred
generally to cold and inaccuracy of diet,
is attacked by symptoms more decidedly febrile or rather inflammatory; rigors, heat, great thirst, pain in the region of the stomach, vomiting by which
green bile and occasionally blood is
thrown up, a loaded yellow tongue,
tension of the hypochondria and costiveness to which succeed bilious and even
bloody discharges. The pain, which has
been described as attended by a remarkable fluttering, has been known to be suddenly translated to the extremities, with

a sort of scorbutic puffiness of the knees,
ancles, and wrists, and a weakness of
the latter resembling the paralysis from
lead. * Petechiæ likewise have made
their appearance with some temporary
relief. † The patient speedily becomes so
feeble and short-breathed, that he can
hardly walk about. The dejection of
spirits is excessive, and the sallow, bloated,
appearance of the skin truly remarkable;
but the body rather emaciates, than swells
greatly; and it is late, before any decided
signs show themselves of accumulations
in the thorax and abdomen. A natural or
increased quantity of urine usually re-
tards these. Hæmorrhages and foul ulcers
are also very apt to occur. Under such
aggravated circumstances, the blood has
been found inflamed; and Dr. Darwin's
authority, already quoted, is very strong in
proving a similar fact. ‡ Altogether these
symptoms have such a resemblance to the
land-scurvy, that I really know no sign by
which they can be distinguished; and I

* Pages 153, 154.   † Pages 153, 155.
‡ Darwin's Zoonomia, vol. i. xxvii. 2.

believe that many of the cases, published under that title, are in fact no other than the disease here described.

The above acute attack of cachexy, if I may use that term, is however comparatively rare. More frequently these signs of an utter depravation of the habit come on in a gradual manner, and with no very sudden exacerbation. They have been in a great measure already enumerated; thirst; habitual fever; loathing of food, with a rotten taste in the mouth; costive but very feeble bowels; dyspnœa on the slightest movement of the body and even on speaking; palpitations; a short cough; swellings of the ancles; emaciation of the rest of the body; a paleness and transparency of complexion, with a pearly colour of the conjunctiva, from which the red vessels disappear, and a death-like paleness of the lips; or a considerable sallowness of skin, with an overflow of bile; urine made rather frequently, particularly at night, and apparently crude, but now and then depositing a bloody sediment. Dropsy generally ensues, unless prevented by diabetes; and the prognosis is unfavourable.

Under such circumstances of impaired digestion and colour, our suspicions are reasonably directed to the viscera of the abdomen. There is not always, however, any decided proof of the exact nature of the injury; and in some instances it seems doubtful, whether the structure of these parts is affected, or only their secretions. That failure of the biliary secretion, which is indicated by a complexion perfectly pale as well as transparent, is a very bad form of the disease. Greater sallowness of colour and an overflow of bile are the evidence of more activity, and permit the use of remedies.

Linnæus has sketched the outlines of this cachectic state with the hand of a master, when in defining it he has used the words, " *pallor corporis œdematosus cum debilitate et mœrore.*" These terms appear to me so descriptive, that I have already quoted them in the former part of this volume, chap. vii., and to that and the succeeding chapter

I beg leave to refer the reader for further observations on this subject and on the purpura or land-scurvy.

As the complaint advances, what are called bilious and rotten sputa are often expectorated. The appearance of these, joined to a peculiarly offensive smell of the breath, has been thought particularly to indicate a schirrus of the liver; but the surface from which they originate has been much mistaken, when it has been supposed that some morbid communication exists between the liver and lungs by adhesion, which furnishes a passage from the former into the bronchia. The dissection recorded in pages 150 and 151 is a sufficient proof, that such sputa may be connected with a scirrhus of that gland, and yet the diaphragm remain sound. Such a communication indeed and a true bilious spitting I believe to be, in this country at least, a very rare occurrence; and I am confident, that the facility with which purulent spittings, attended by bilious symptoms, are called hepatic, is the source of infinite mischief by appearing to justify, what can rarely be justified in internal ulcers, a mercurial course.

The anasarca during courses of mercury, when sudden and connected with cold, has nothing in it very untractable; but if it rises gradually and from the repeated introduction of that poison into the system, it is a truly formidable disease. The natural and animal functions suffer a remarkable depression, whilst on the contrary the movement of the heart and arteries is carried on with a degree of tension peculiar to that state. The blood is not only unusually cupped; but the buff has been known to form, where it has only trickled down the arm; and the occasional whiteness both of that crust and of the serum are deserving of much notice. When this distemper has proceeded to a great extent, it is hardly cured.

The common symptomatic swellings are sometimes converted into this by mercury given for the relief of the obstructions; and then nothing favourable is to be expected.

The mercurial hectic in syphilis, which puts, or ought to put, an instant stop to the use of that mineral, I have known once or twice to be distinguished by a serous state of the urine, even though there has been no absolute anasarca. How far this sign prevails generally, it is very important to enquire; since we frequently want all the evidence which the nature of the subject will admit, with regard to the propriety of continuing a mercurial course.

SECTION III.

Of the Hydrothorax, or Dropsy of the Cavities of the Thorax and Pericardium.

THE hydrothorax, as has been already observed, is not an unusual termination of diffused dropsies. Sometimes the chest is attacked in the first place.

This occurs in old and weak subjects, and is attended generally by signs of broken health, particularly a pale sallow complexion. The anasarca increases gradually; and in the early stage I have known it to be absolutely wanting. There is usually a short cough, and something so far febrile about such patients, that they are hurt by whatever has a tendency to excite inflammation. Often, upon recollection, they are able to trace their symptoms, or at least the sudden increase of them, to some imprudent exposure in bad weather; and they are particularly sensible to the effects both of cold and of close rooms. The urine gives a loose and slight coagulum, and is often loaded with a red sediment. In these cases particularly, gout thrown to the extremities is wont to give a great and unexpected relief.

There is another form of hydrothorax, which may occur at a less advanced age, and is a true example of dropsical inflammation. Serum and lymph are thrown out instead of pus. There is even a partial suppuration of the lung. That organ becomes at length compressed and greatly diminished in bulk ; and life is extinguished by this mechanical violence. Who, that has witnessed a dissection under such circumstances, but must acknowledge, how much our art might have done in preventing this accumulation, how little in removing it ? *

This variety is, I believe, sometimes accompanied by a pain or numbness and œdema of the arm on the affected side † ; in the former, both arms are thought occasionally to sympathize.

* Chapter IX. case I. see also page 96.
† Page 172.

The principal signs of water in the cavities of the thorax or pericardium are, a more than ordinary dyspnœa particularly marked on going up hill, an irregular or intermittent pulse, a difficulty of lying down in bed, frightful dreams, as of drowning or falling down a precipice, from which the patient awakes agitated to the most distressing suffocations with palpitations of the heart, and a sense of fluctuation observed by the patient himself.

These signs are not, in strict propriety, pathognomic. All of them, excepting the last, occasionally attend other disorders; all, but the first, may be absent in this. And yet there are combinations of them, the evidence of which it is hardly possible to resist.

To prove the uncertainty of these signs, singly considered, it is only necessary to state that the pulse is rendered irregular by organic injuries of the heart, and it is sometimes perfectly regular in the most decided hydrothorax. *

Again, the orthopnœa is often an asthma-

* Cases and Dissections, pages 107 and 163.

tic symptom; and I have known persons prefer the horizontal posture in bed, in whom dissection, or other conclusive evidence, proved that an hydrothorax existed. *

Similar assertions may be made of the hurried dreams and nightly suffocations. †

Of the fluctuation observed by the practitioner I have no experience. That complained of now and then by the patient is seated, as far as I have been able to learn, at the lower part of the sternum on the left side. It may be supposed to be exaggerated by his fears; yet more than one very calm person has assured me of its reality. ‡ Hypochondriacs and dyspeptics have sometimes complained of a similar feeling; and the opinion of its being connected with the presence of water has taken firm possession of them. When combined, however, with other evidence, and in persons of sober judgment, it is of great weight. I believe it belongs more to the dropsy of the pericardium, than of the cavities of the thorax; as indeed its situation implies.

* Case and Dissection, page 104; Case, page 57.
† Case and Dissection, pages 47 and 104; Case, p. 57.
‡ Cases, pages 57 and 172.

And if there are any other circumstances which should direct our attention particularly to the former of these, they are, a remarkable sense of faintness, combining itself with the dyspnœa produced by exercise * and change of position † ; and in bed, even when difficulty of breathing is present, the preference of a posture different from the erect, as of the completely horizontal ‡, or a considerable inclination forwards, the face nearly resting on the knees. §

The distressing dreams and nightly suffocations I consider to be very rarely indeed absent, where the water presses on the lungs.

A remarkable dyspnœa is present in all, not only increased on going up stairs, but attended by an embarrassed gait, a loaded countenance, an habitual slowness and pause in speaking, a peculiar look of distress,

---

* Page 57.   † Page 107, line 9.

‡ Case, p. 57 ; Case and Dissection, page 104 ; and Maclean on Hydrothorax, pages 68 and 69.

§ In a patient at St. Bartholomew's Hospital, who could bear no other posture in bed than the leaning forwards and resting on his knees, I found after death the pericardium containing half a pint of clear serum, the membranes not apparently inflamed, lungs sound, and no water in the cavities of the thorax.

not easy to describe, and from which the features rarely return to their proper harmony, even though the patient obtain relief.

On the whole, so remote from entire certainty are these signs, that in one in whom all, except the sense of fluctuation, were combined, with some others indeed super-added, a pulse every way irregular, palpitations, cough, dyspnœa, inability of remaining in the bed for a single instant, suffocations and deliquia after sleeping even in his chair, and an anxious embarrassed countenance, the whole injury was found, on dissection, to be seated in the body of the lung, and the lymphatic glands at its root. *

We can hardly expect that the signs of diseased organization, which in fact are nothing but impeded functions, should be as various as the disorganizations themselves; still less that, complicated as these injuries often are and modified by the sensibility of the subject, the symptoms peculiar to each, even if there be any such, should always be

* Case, page 47.

Q 2

able to develope themselves.   A probability short of certainty must regulate our
decision.   If to many of the signs above
described be added a dropsical habit with
a serous condition of the urine, the existence of an hydrothorax will be in the
highest degree probable ; if the patient has
been before relieved by diuretics, it can no
longer admit of doubt.

Are a dyspnœa and orthopnœa of a few
days duration, and a highly serous condition of the urine, without any sort of dropsy
besides to account for it, sufficient evidence
of a dropsy existing in the chest ? *

Anasarca of the lungs does not appear to
be very common.   Dr. Baillie never met
with a satisfactory case of it on dissection † ;
which argues that its frequency in the living body is over-rated, or that it is not a
fatal disorder.   At least its symptoms, as
distinguished from hydrothorax, are not
sufficiently understood.

* See Case III. pages 167 and 168.
† Baillie's Morbid Anatomy, Appendix, p. 21.

SECTION IV.

Of the Ascites, or Dropsy of the Belly, and of the Tympany.

THE ascites does not demand much separate consideration. Its presence is detected by what is called the sense of fluctuation, or the shock communicated to the hand held on one side of the abdomen, whilst an impetus is given to its contents by a gentle blow on the other side. This sensation of a fluid is peculiar and well understood by those who have once experienced it. It is decidedly different from the elastic vibration and hollow sound communicated by air pent up in the stomach or intestines, which likewise gives a remarkable sense of lightness hardly to be expected in a tumour of so much bulk, a feeling so obvious to the mere touch, that there can be no necessity for the experiment of weighing the patient, suggested by Van Swieten. *

In the last stage of general dropsy, a tympany has been observed, and has even succeeded to the ascites. It is principally seated in the region of the stomach ; and after death, besides the general flatulency of the intestines, that organ has been found enormously distended with air, which was inflammable and not the fixed, as it has been usually asserted to be.† This circumstance should have been expressed in the relation of the morbid appearances, pages 109 and 164, amongst which it certainly was observed.

I have been surprised at the long period, many weeks, during which the stomach has

* Vide Van Swieten Commentaria, tom. iv. p. 172. " Præcipua signa sunt, si abdomen percussum instar " tympani resonet, et si æger ad stateram levis sit, cum " e contra in ascite ægri ob collectam aquam pondus " insigne habeant."

† Dr. Baillie, speaking of air in the intestines after death, says, " this air probably differs somewhat at dif- " ferent times; in several trials which I have made, it " never showed signs of containing any proportion of " inflammable, but always a very sensible proportion " of fixed air." — Morbid Anatomy, p. 129.

10

continued thus distended and apparently unfit for any process of digestion, and yet life has been protracted.* Two striking instances of it, one in particular in a hospital in London, followed the use of digitalis, which had operated beneficially with regard to the swellings, but had greatly debilitated the nerves. Whether this result can be at all the effect of the remedy as well as of the disease, is a grave consideration.

These accumulations are sometimes so combined, as to confuse the sensation resulting from each. But any nice discrimination will be of less consequence in such a state, where an operation cannot be advisable.

A sero-purulent fluid filling the cavity of the abdomen, and without any anasarea or even bloated appearance of the skin, has been attended by some albumen in the urine.† This circumstance I consider of no slight importance in explaining the real nature of that impregnation.

* Page 164.   † Page 181.

Q 4

SECTION V.

Of the Hydrocephalus Internus, or Dropsy of the Ventricles of the Brain.

THE hydrocephalus has been described in pages 209 and 212, as far as I have found it to be attended by a coagulable state of the urine. The dropsical metastases to and from the brain, mentioned by authors, appear to be of this nature, as are probably all those cases which occur after scarlatina. But I suspect that hydrocephalus originates much less frequently in this constitutional dropsy, than in other causes to which the character above alluded to does not belong. So much the more discouraging will be the aspect of the disease. That remarkable sign denotes a specific error in the constitution, and has appropriate remedies ; whilst the obscurity of its other causes leaves much to conjecture, and when the disease is established, but little to hope.

Can there be a more humiliating picture of the state of medical opinion on this subject, and of the value of medical conclusions, than the following extracts from an author of approved credit on the disorders of children, Dr. Underwood?

Page 280. " Though I have made men-
" tion of mercury," says he, " I cannot say I
" have seen any decidedly good effects from
" its use, either as a purge or an altera-
" tive, (when the disease has been clearly
" ascertained,) administered either exter-
" nally or internally, though I have had
" recourse to it very early as well as late in
" the disease."

Page 281. " It is proper to observe, that
" mercury has been strongly recommended
" by Drs. Carmichael Smith, Dobson, John
" Hunter, Haygarth, Moseley, and Dr.
" Armstrong; but I am informed by other
" physicians of eminence, that they have
" not been so successful in the use of it."

Page 284. " Dr. Percival recommends
" joining the digitalis with opium and ca-
" lomel; though he is inclined to think

" that the good effects produced by this
" composition are rather attributable to
" the combination of the opium and calo-
" mel, than to the digitalis."

> *Page 285.* " Dr. Temple was led to ad-
" vise the doronicum germanicum in hy-
" drocephalus, and in a recent instance
" with marked success, in consequence of
" an abundant perspiration from the head.
" Opium and calomel were indeed joined
" with it ; but as it is not known that such
" effects have been produced from the
" combination of mercury and opium, he
" concludes that the doronicum had a con-
" siderable share in them."

What can the reader conclude, but that
nothing is known of this disease, and that
the most powerful instruments are wielded
in the dark ?

SECTION VI.

Of the Diabetes Serosus, or an excessive Discharge of Serous Urine.

IN some cases, the quantity of urine is so much increased, as to give suspicion of a diabetes. The swellings are in a great measure prevented by this excessive discharge; but no other benefit is derived from it. On the contrary, the system is evidently more embarrassed by the loss of serum, than it would have been even by its accumulation. There is a burning thirst, with fever, dry skin, and rapid emaciation of the whole body. The nerves in particular are greatly affected; the despondency being extreme, and the fretfulness of mind often unconquerable by any effort of reason.

More urine is evacuated in the night than in the day; and the urinary organs themselves sometimes suffer from a feebleness and irritation, similar to what have been observed in the diabetes mellitus.

Of the proportional frequency with which these two species occur, I am unable to make a correct estimate. I believe that the former to a certain degree is the more common, but that the quantity discharged in it is never so preternaturally excessive, as in the latter, in which, as we are informed, it has amounted to 12 quarts, to 27 pounds, and even 36 pounds daily.*

The descriptions of this disease given by the ancients have been general, and have contained no allusion to these qualities of the urine. They have, nevertheless, been considered to relate to the diabetes melli tus almost exclusively, with what justice, may be well doubted. The noted expression used by some of these physicians, *hydrops ad matulam*, is exactly descriptive of the serous diabetes ; and many remarks of Aretæus are applicable to it only.

In his detail of the symptoms †, that author dwells principally on the extreme

* Rollo on Diabetes, pages 17. 160. 169.
† Aretæus de Morbis Diuturnis, lib. ii. cap. ii.

thirst, common to both species, and wholly omits to notice the boulimy or inordinate appetite, which forms so striking a feature of the diabetes mellitus, but is often changed to a loathing of food in the serous. His chapter on the cure he commences by stating*, that diabetes is a species of dropsy, both in its cause and its general nature, and differs from it only in the channel by which the humours pass out of the circulation ; that in dropsy they are deposited at rest in the cavities of the body, in diabetes are carried off by the kidneys and bladder. He adds, that if relief is obtained in dropsy, it is by that channel, namely, the urinary organs ; but that this relief consists rather in the solution of the cause, than in the mere removal of the burthen.

The regimen and diet, and in a great measure even the medical remedies, he directs to be nearly the same in both, and particularly recommends in diabetes the use of sweet and astringent wines. This recommendation, if it proceeded from any expe-

* Aretæus de Curat. Diuturn. lib. ii. cap. ii.

rience of their utility, and not from a mere theoretical notion, must have been directed against the dropsical excess of urine principally. And it is worthy of remark, that Sydenham, when he prescribes sweet wines in diabetes, appears to have had in his more immediate contemplation that which occurred in elderly persons after intermittents, no doubt connected with a dropsical habit.*

It is difficult to view those doctrines of Aretæus, illustrated as they are by the facts contained in this volume, in any other light than as evidences that he drew his descriptions from the serous as well as the saccharine diabetes.

Dr. Heberden's opinion is very similar to that above quoted. Speaking of the excess of urine, and of the intense thirst which usually precedes it : " I have hardly," says he, " known them but in very infirm and " old people, in whom age or distemper had " so far injured some of the parts necessary " to life, that death must soon have ensued, " whether the patient made too much water

* Sydenhami Opera, p. 307.

" and was wasted in a diabetes, or made
" hardly any, and was bloated in a dropsy.
" It is not very improbable that some tri-
" vial circumstance determined the body
" to take on one of these two diseases rather
" than the other, and that the removing of
" either of them would do but little to-
" wards saving the patient's life." *

If the ancients have overlooked the composition of the urine in these excessive discharges, more modern writers have been
not wholly free from the same neglect, and
have often confounded, under the term
diabetes insipidus, all those cases in which
the sweet taste was not detected.

The more accurate practice of evaporation lately adopted has accidentally eluci-
dated this subject, and shows in a strong
point of view what great discoveries labour
and accident may yet make in the history
of diseases.

Dr. Latham, on evaporating the urine of
a suspected diabetic patient, observed a
large quantity of albumen. Mr. Watts of
Glasgow, under similar circumstances, de-

* Heberden's Commentaries, chap. xxvi. Diabetes.

tected the same substance in a much larger proportion.

Cases of it less severe and obscured by the presence of anasarca not uncommonly occur. Stimulating diuretics have appeared to me to produce it. I have less hesitation in saying, that mercury has that effect; and the state of the kidneys in two dissections, after excessive mercurial courses*, would induce a belief, that it is not wholly unconnected with a local affection of those glands.

The saccharine and serous diabetes may perhaps be combined; and the quantity of serum present may possibly conceal the sweetness of the taste. Mr. Watts of Glasgow, in the case before mentioned, where the urine was insipid, first obtained by heat a large coagulum, and then by evaporating the strained fluid, an unusual proportion of extractive matter, which when treated with nitrous acid and water, afforded a considerable quantity of oxalic acid.†

There is likewise something remarkable

* Pages 109 and 184.
† Watts on Diabetes, p. 74.

in the quality which albuminous urine, when pale and copious, has been found to possess, of continuing long without any decomposition, and even reddening for an unusual period the vegetable blues. This character, however, is by no means constant. And altogether the subject is so new, as rather to demand further investigation than to require or even permit any general conclusions at present.

R

CHAPTER XIV.

THE SAME SUBJECT CONTINUED.

SECTION I.

Of the Remote Causes.

THE predisposition to this disease consists
principally of a certain feebleness and inactivity of constitution, called the phlegmatic temperament.   Its signs are well
understood, and it is beyond any doubt hereditary.   On this account dropsy itself
has been called an hereditary disorder; and
it certainly is so, in the only sense in which
any disease is entitled to that appellation.
This opinion has always been very prevalent; of which a stronger proof can hardly
be adduced, than the superstitious ceremo-

nies alluded to by Van Swieten. He states on the authority of Plutarch, that, amongst the ancients, the children of those who died consumptive or dropsical sat with their feet immersed in water, whilst the dead bodies were burnt, that the disease might not pass to them; and from Van Helmont, that, in Antwerp, the vulgar thought the dropsy would descend to the next heir, unless all the water was drawn off from the dead body.*

The same feebleness of constitution is artificially produced by poor diet, bad air, the depressing passions, and large evacuations of any kind, particularly great losses of blood.

Some of these are undoubtedly exciting causes likewise; but as with the debility essential to the disease there is often combined in the present form an inflammation from the very commencement, so some of its exciting causes will be found to partake of this latter character.

The gout is probably both a predisposing and exciting cause. Frequent paroxysms of

* Van Swieten, Commentaria, tom. iv. p. 192.

R 2

it, particularly if they are ever retrocedent, bring on a dangerous feebleness of the habit ; whilst the sudden accumulations on the chest, which occur in such subjects not without some obscure signs of inflammation appear to resemble a misplaced gout.

Some of the most remarkable of the other causes are, as follows :

Scarlatina. —— There is something hitherto obscure in the disposition to œdematous swellings which scarlatina leaves. The time, the symptoms, and subjects of this attack, by no means permit the opinion that it originates in mere debility. On the contrary the attendants are often persuaded, that the patient has caught some fresh cold ; and it is certainly not improbable, that the previous irritation and inflammation of the skin may be followed by an opposite state of it, incapable of supporting even the common changes of temperature.

This doctrine is strongly supported by M. Meglie, in the Journal de Médicine, Jan. 1811. He thinks that sudden changes from a hot to a cold temperature, and even the contrary, are the exciting causes of the scarlatinous anasarca; that in order to avoid it, it is proper to submit to the most rigid confinement, in the winter for about six weeks, and that during this period tender children should not place themselves too near even to a closed window.

The obscurity however, above alluded-to, refers only to the origin of the complaint; in its symptoms, it is the plainest possible specimen of the disease of which I am treating, a sort of epitome of the dropsical habit, which at other times we find complicated and confused by a variety of extraneous circumstances.

The abuse of mercury. — The effects of mercurial courses badly conducted are very severe, but of a character not hitherto entirely understood. By some authors they have been thought inflammatory, by others a disease in which loss of tone predominates; and it is not unreasonable to suppose that they do actually vary in these respects. The predisposition and habits of the patient may determine much; the feebleness of particular organs often fixes the part, on which the principal violence of the distemper is to be exerted; whilst we must refer somewhat to the mode in which that poison has reached the circulation, to the effect which it has produced on the discharges, particularly those of the intestines, and to the causes that may have prevented its proper excretion. Thus it is probable that if calomel has been chosen and a diarrhœa has followed its repeated use, the mercurial habit, that ultimately ensues, will be blended with much weakness ; whilst if the mercury has been passed by the absorbents of the skin, and no great discharges have taken place, or the secretions have been checked by cold, a disorder will follow more distinguished by inflammation than debility.

Mr. Mathias has made some very excellent remarks on the mercurial habit. The irritation produced by that mineral he considers to be of a very inflammatory kind, adding, that the blood is found buffed in a remarkable degree ; and that venæsection is the best remedy even for a salivation. *

A physician, who had great opportunities of witnessing the use of mercury, Dr.

Mathias on the Mercurial Disease.

Paisley, thus expresses himself with regard to its effects even in a hot climate. " It " is too apt to leave behind it an inflam- " matory diathesis, so much so indeed, " that I would recommend to you as a " general rule in all severe attacks of dis- " ease, where mercury has preceded, to " bleed early and freely. For watching, " fatigues, and bodily exercise of the se- " verest kinds have not greater effects in " wasting the thinner parts of the blood, " and producing a density of it, than mer- " curial courses." *

These remarks deserve much attention, if we would ascertain the nature of the common mercurial habit; they apply like-wise in a great degree to the dropsy from the same cause. No stronger examples indeed of inflammation can be adduced, than some of the cases of it described in this volume. That such a disposition ex-tends to them all, I by no means assert; and still further, if the symptoms, related in pages 34 and 35, are rightly attributed

* Curtis's Diseases of India, p. 371. Letter from Dr. Paisley.

to mercury, it would appear that even the serous state of the urine is not uniformly present. *

There is a species of dropsical accumulation, which is so constantly treated by mercury, that I know not if I shall obtain from every reader an acknowledgment, that mercury may possibly bring it on. It appears to me, however, that no accidents proper to the disease can account for all those fatal conversions to the head, which of late years have so frequently taken place in the fevers of children ; and I have on some occasions been disposed to attribute them to excessive and repeated doses of calomel, which either not moving the bowels, as was expected, have given evidence of being absorbed, or on the other hand have purged too violently and been succeeded by a diarrhœa without bile, and a prostration of strength from which the little patient has never risen. Its less se-

* Dr. Wells's observations on the effects of Mercury are of importance in this question. He has proved decidedly, that salivations have a great tendency to produce a serous state of the urine, but that this effect is not uniform.

13

vere effects are sometimes of no slight importance, a slow and imperfect recovery, a languid feverish habit, and a disposition to scrophula. It need not surprise us, that in children this disposition, particularly if so excited, should often fall on the part most liable to every impression, and most actively developing itself, the brain; since even in adults, mercury is inimical to the nervous system. Parents have something to regret, who are so perpetually giving calomel to their own children, without any distinction or care, as a common domestic remedy. And it is difficult to conceive on what view of the subject even practitioners proceed, who indulge in its use with less scruple than ever, with less attention as to dose, with less caution as to management, whilst they are observing and lamenting the daily increasing ravages of hereditary scrophulous disorders. It can hardly be in the present day from want of calomel, that such a taint is propagated. Altogether the excellence of this remedy in many, even infantile, cases, its cleansing powers, its inflammatory and its debilitating action, render it a two-edged sword.

The drinking too freely of cold liquors when heated ; and the external application of cold. —— Boerhaave's Aphorism is very minute with regard to the former of these. *Potus nimius frigidæ subitus, neque vomitu, neque alvo, neque sudore, vel urina, calore motuve excitatis, excretus.* * The ancient physicians mention the same fact ; and Van Swieten asserts that, in soldiers on a march exhausted by heat and fatigue, he has known the drinking of cold water bring on, in some instances, a fatal pleurisy, in others, a dropsy. † The relation, which these two diseases here bear to each other, is very worthy of remark.

I have sometimes witnessed similar effects from large quantities of weak and cold cider, drunk by labourers in the harvest in this county ; and there is a saying almost proverbial amongst them, that when the cider falls into their legs, the fox-glove, called by them, cow-flop, carries it off.

If cold acting on the stomach is capable of producing dropsy as well as pleurisy,

---

* Boerhaave's Aphorism, 1229.

† Van Swieten, Commentaria, tom. iv. page 192.

there seems to be no reason for denying, that it may do the same when applied to the surface of the body; although, from finding internal inflammations to be so much more common a consequence of taking cold, authors have in some measure overlooked the anasarca arising from the same cause.

Of the fact, however, little doubt can be entertained. There is even some reason to think, that the swellings after scarlatina are partly referrible to cold acting on a tender and denuded skin. And the comparative rareness of the diffused dropsy in very hot climates, which has been asserted on good authority, proves, if true, its great connection with a low temperature and obstructed perspiration.

The improper exhibition of bark and steel.—These remedies on many occasions have greatly aggravated the disorder; sometimes they have appeared to produce it, or at least have first made it evident.

Stahl's remarks on this subject, in his article *De Hydrope*, are worth consulting.

Topical injuries and inflammations of the limbs.—Dr. Monro mentions a man who, in consequence of a sprain of the wrist from lifting a great weight, became completely anasarcous. * The wrist immediately swelled, and the swelling spread from thence all over his body. † Such an instance is probably very rare, nor should I have alluded to it here, but as it seems to bear some analogy to that swelling of one leg, mentioned pages 124 and 126, from which, as from a point, the œdema spread universally. ‡

This list of causes might perhaps be increased by the addition of some acuté disorders : I am unwilling, however, to assert more than I have seen.

But the most important and most fatal of all agents, in producing this complaint, still remains to be mentioned, an unsoundness of the digestive organs, which impairs the nourishment of the body, vitiates the

---

* Such an exciting cause would argue the effusion to arise, not from mere weakness, but from inflammation ; and no doubt the cellular membrane would, if examined, exhibit appearances of this kind.

† Monro on Dropsy, page 10.   Note.

‡ See also page 87.

blood, and gives vigour and operation to every other cause.

The free use of spirituous liquors greatly contributes to such an incurable taint, and independently of that effect has been thought by many physicians capable of exciting a true dropsy.

SECTION II.

Of the Appearances on Dissection.

The information afforded by dissections has hitherto been very imperfect ; but the novelty and importance of the subject render all observations of this kind in some degree valuable. I shall briefly recapitulate them :

I. Case, page 94, of a woman, who, after recovering from scarlatinous dropsy and pain of the side, died in consequence of a caries of the os sacrum. The pleura of the left lung covered with coagulated lymph, in a spot answering to the seat of the pain; immediately under that membrane, and separating it from the lung, a small abscess; other parts nearly natural.

II. Case, page 104; supposed to originate in the excessive use of mercury; remarkable for very inflammatory symptoms, urine highly serous, a tense sore œdema moving from one part of the body to another, a pulse by no means interrupted, a preference of the horizontal posture, and the most excessive loss of strength and spirits. Pericardium much inflamed, containing three ounces of a turbid whitish fluid; pleura somewhat inflamed, in each cavity from ten to twelve ounces of fluid; stomach greatly distended with air, which, on applying a lighted candle to an opening made in it, burnt with a deep blue flame, till the stomach entirely collapsed; slight marks of inflammation and adhesions about the peritonæum; liver rather firmer than ordinary; kidneys unusually solid, and containing two or three small hydatids; an ounce of water in each lateral ventricle of the brain; cellular membrane of the whole body, particularly the loins, presenting an unusual resistance to the knife, and containing an effusion somewhat transparent and coagulated; fluid, which drained off, coagulating spontaneously on exposure to air.

III. Case, page 181, of a woman, who had undergone enormous courses of mercury, even whilst pregnant, and was also very intemperate. Liver greatly enlarged and hardened; kidneys likewise large and hard, and their structure confused, particularly in respect to the distinction between the cortical and medullary part.

IV. Case, page 115, distinguished by a remarkable diarrhœa, for the cure of which mercury had been vainly used. Ulcers of the cæcum and colon; kidneys remarkably loaded with blood; lungs filled with tubercles.

V. Case, page 132, attributed to cold. Thorax and abdomen healthy, except that in the former, there was an appearance, rather recent, of the adhesive inflammation; in the head, an aneurism of the basilary artery; and the ventricles filled with coagulated blood; cellular membrane unusually firm, and containing an effusion similar to that described, No. II. The bursting of this aneurism had been the cause of the fatal attack, which in its symptoms greatly resembled hydrocephalus internus.

VI. Case, page 149, under the article cachexy, distinguished by a whey-coloured urine and sanious sputa. Lower part of the right lung loaded with coagula of blood; liver scirrhous; diaphragm perfectly free; membranes of the brain inflamed, half an ounce of water in each ventricle.

VII. Case, page 164, a regular pulse, abdomen tympanitic for some weeks before death. Right side of the thorax filled with water, in which flakes of lymph swam; lung compressed to the size of a man's fist; under its membrane a small abscess; pleura pulmonalis, on both sides of the thorax, covered with a thick coat of lymph; stomach greatly distended with air, which on trial proved wholly inflammable; liver rather large and firm; kidneys very small and sound, excepting two or three hydatids.

VIII. Case, page 189, of a boy, in whom the urine, in a fever, under the use of very large doses of calomel, became loaded with a fœtid bloody sediment. Ventricles of the brain distended with water, signs of inflammation on their surfaces, as well as on the pia mater.

IX. Case (for which see the postscript) of a young man, in whom the disease, a general anasarca, was apparently brought on by cold and exposure to rain, and proved rapidly fatal by the spreading of an erysipelas on the integuments of the chest and abdomen. The pleuræ inflamed and covered almost universally with an adventitious lymphy membrane ; cellular membrane loaded with water, and with a soft, gelatinous, imperfectly coagulated effusion, interspersed with spots of blood, opposite to the inflamed surface on the skin. Viscera nearly sound.

The lymphatic vessels are found unusually thickened and distended in dropsical bodies ; so that such subjects are much preferred for anatomical preparations. This appears to be a state similar to the dilatation and thickening of varicose veins, indicating inactivity and consequent accumulation.

The serum of the cavities in this disease

s

possesses various degrees of dilution ; the fluid drawn off by tapping in the ascites, has resembled soapy water, and that not once only, but after repeated operations* ; and what is discharged by scarifications is almost aqueous.

The following remarks occur to me from the preceding statement : —

1st. That the urinary organs are often free from any appearance of unsound structure, notwithstanding the great fault in their secretion.

2d. That in two mercurial cases, the kidneys were firmer than ordinary, in one of them very strikingly so, approaching to scirrhus ; but whether this is merely accidental, or the effect of such a course, and what relation it bears to the discharge of serum, must be left for future observation.†

3d. That an unhealthy state of the liver is likewise not an uncommon morbid appearance ; in two instances out of eight it was scirrhous, in one of these greatly en-

---

* Page 122.

† In a dissection related by Dr. Wells, for which see the postscript, the kidneys were found thickened and confused in their structure.

larged; in a third, harder than ordinary; and in a fourth, rather large and firm.

4th. That an inflammatory state of some serous membrane, particularly the pleura, is frequent, producing the effusion of a serous fluid, which is more opaque and lymphy, and the membrane more disfigured, in proportion to the signs of general inflammation and of local pain, and the firmness and quantity of coagulum in the urine.

5th. That where on the surface of the pleura pulmonalis lymph has been thrown out, true pus has sometimes been deposited between it and the lung; and a purulent expectoration has been often so marked during life, that it is beyond any doubt, large abscesses would have been found in the lungs on dissection.

6th. Some attention is due to the state of the cellular membrane described in three cases, No. II. No. V. and No. IX. The appearances No. II. were truly remarkable, and answered exactly to the signs, that had prevailed during life, of a sort of inflammatory anasarca, not distinguished by any redness of the surface, but a tension and soreness and puffy swelling passing from

s 2

one part to another, as if the cellular membrane under the skin had been affected
with an erysipelas. A coagulating effusion,
apparently of a gelatinous nature, is, I
believe, not very uncommon in anasarca;
and it does not seem to be ascertained,
whether or not this coagulation has taken
place during life. It may not be improper
here to mention, that in those painful swellings of the lower extremities, which occur
mostly after pregnancy, the urine, though
often scanty, is not coagulable.

Lastly, whilst in these anatomical observations we find varieties of injury, in the
head, thorax, abdomen, and even cellular
membrane, we must not forget to add to
the account those perfect recoveries which
prove the occasional mildness of the disease,
and the little mischief which any of these
parts have sustained.

SECTION III.

Of the proximate Cause.

THE proximate cause of dropsy has hitherto received no satisfactory explanation. In health, the absorption keeps pace with the secretion, and permits sufficient vapour only to moisten the surfaces. All accumulation therefore is disease, and beyond any doubt it must immediately proceed from a secretion greater than the absorption. But to produce this excess, is the secretion positively increased, or the absorption diminished, or both? If the former, is it produced by a laxity of the exhalant vessels, that characteristic of the hydropic diathesis as Dr. Cullen thinks *, or by their greater activity? If the latter, is the absorbent system in a torpid state, or labouring under a morbid irritability and stricture? †

* Cullen's First Lines, vol. iv. page 261.
‡ Maclean on Hydrothorax, pages 250, 253, &c.

An impoverished condition of the blood likewise has been thought to give a tendency to aqueous effusions. Is it impossible, that an altered texture of that fluid, different from mere thinness, and disposing it speedily to separate into its constituent parts, may have the same effect?

Neither is it to be forgotten, that absorption may be diminished not merely by a fault of the absorbent vessels, but of the secretion presented to them, different from the natural and not suited to their elective powers.

Writers in general, observing the weakness of the habit in this disease, have inclined to the opinion, that it is immediately produced by a loss of strength and firmness in the parts concerned, a laxity of the exhalant system, an inactivity of the absorbents, and a watery state of the blood.

Some of the appearances however, I speak particularly of the dropsy with coagulable urine, are not favourable to the uniform truth at least of this opinion.

1st. The serum of the affected cavities has been often found opaque in various degrees, discoloured, and containing pieces of lymph; and in one instance even the fluid of the cellular membrane coagulated spontaneously. This very variety proves a morbid state; and there can be no doubt, that it sometimes tends towards the inflammatory.

Even where the contained fluid is more clear and diluted, and only partially coagulates by heat and acids, it is very difficult to determine in what respects it differs from the healthy secretion. The minute quantity of the latter, and the great difference between the dead and the living body, render all such comparisons imperfect and inconclusive.

The ancients, not without much propriety, termed the natural secretion an exhalation. Mr. John Hunter asserts, that the juices which lubricate surfaces are in a volatile state while the animal is alive.

Dr. Darwin goes so far as to assert, that the property of coagulation by heat is acquired by stagnation only. *

Dr. Baillie considers, that no decisive trials have been, or, from the very nature

---

* Darwin's Zoonomia, vol. i. sect. xxix. 4.

of the subject, can be made, unless on the contents of the ventricles of the brain, where some water is usually found even in the healthy condition of that organ. *

Mr. Hewson is considered by many persons to have decided the nature of this secretion. By gently scraping the surfaces of the cavities with a wet tea-spoon, in animals recently killed, he collected fluid sufficient for experiment, and ascertained the following qualities of it ; that on being suffered to rest, exposed to the air, it jellies in about half an hour, less firmly in young and weak animals, than in old and strong ones, and requires a longer time for that process, where the animal has been reduced to great weakness, although the blood under the same circumstances coagulates sooner ; that it resembles in every respect the fluid found in the lymphatics, and approaches to the coagulable lymph.†

---

* Baillie's Morbid Anatomy, pages 304 and 305.

† By the term jellying, the author probably means no more than spontaneous coagulation; since he applies the same word to the lymph of the blood, and it does not at all appear that any experiments were made

His conclusions from these observations, as applied to disease, are, that this healthy lymph is a mean between the fluid of dropsy and the coagulated membranes of inflammation. The former he asserts to be so diluted as not to coagulate but by heat and acids, being a serum only; the latter to be a lymph altered to the contrary extreme of rapid coagulation, and showing itself in inflammatory crusts; and that pus, in a still higher degree of inflammation, is sometimes secreted by the same vessels. *

These experiments are, no doubt, faithfully made, and come from very considerable authority; but they seem liable to many objections, arising from the mode in which the fluid was collected, and the fallacy of reasoning from the dead to the living body, from other animals to the human subject. Nor should it be overlooked, that all the observations relating to the healthy state are derived from the former, to the diseased, from the latter.

to ascertain its properties with regard to heat, re-solution in warm water, &c.

* Hewson on the Blood, vol. ii. page 103.

Without laying too much stress on these difficulties, it is, however, remarkable, that the comparative experiments least liable to objection, in the human subject alone, furnish conclusions very opposite to those of Mr. Hewson. Dr. Baillie states, as the result of his own observations, that the water of hydrocephalus is less diluted, and discovers more animal matter by the common tests, than the contents of the same cavities, when there has been no previous affection of the head. * Still further, the only example of spontaneous coagulation of the cellular serum has been in a case of anasarca † ; in the same state of disease, the cells have been loaded with an effusion imperfectly coagulated and lymphy, as well as with a fluid ; in some a floating lymph has been observed, mixed with a diluted serum ‡ ; even the membranes have been covered with an inflammatory crust, whilst there has been a true dropsy of the cavity. § These are specimens of disease, which Mr. Hewson's doctrine would prove

* Baillie's Morbid Anatomy, pages 304 and 305.
† Page 110. ‡ Pages 109, 129, &c. § Page 165, &c.

to involve a contradiction in terms, a dropsical inflammation.

Mr. Hunter's experiments set in its true light a circumstance, rather overlooked probably than denied in such inquiries, that the fluids which lubricate surfaces are in some degree volatile; and that, as the living principle departs, this quality disappears likewise. His own words will best illustrate his opinion.

" Some of the juices of a living animal,
" whether circulating, or out of circula-
" tion, as those which lubricate surfaces,
" are in a volatile state while the animal is
" alive; for when the scarfskin is taken
" off, the part soon dries; and if the skin
" is removed from a newly killed animal,
" it immediately dries; or if a cavity is
" opened, the surface of the cavity dries
" quickly; this shows that some part of
" the juices must have evaporated from the
" surface: but let the animal cool before
" it is skinned, or the cavity is opened,
" and then give it the same degree of heat
" that it had when alive, you will find, on
" taking off the skin, no immediate sensi-
" ble evaporation; but the part so expos-

" ed will remain moist.   This volatility I
" conceive therefore to be connected with
" life, and not with the circulation ; for
" that is stopped in both cases before the
" experiment.   Whether it is this volatile
" part that gives the smell that most re-
" cently killed animals have upon being
" skinned, or opened, I do not know ;
" but it may be observed, that it follows
" the same rules ; for if the animal is
" allowed to cool, it loses this smell,
" although warmed to the same degree of
" heat as when alive." *

The solid part then of these secretions
appears, in the healthy state, to be held in
a very fine solution, of which the term,
watery, gives us no correct idea.   In the
disease of which we are treating, they are
probably thrown out in a less subtle and
elaborate form ; what other changes take
place in the proportion of coagulable
matter, and its disposition to separate, is
involved in great doubt ; but it may be a
guide to us in so difficult an inquiry to
recollect, that in some instances of dropsy

* Hunter on the Blood, pages 36 and 37.

the effusion undoubtedly contains a portion of coagulating lymph, and seems to be in its very essence inflammatory.

2. In addition to those appearances of the dropsical fluid, which argue a secretion often different from that of mere relaxation, the membranes likewise are sometimes greatly inflamed and disfigured; instances of which may be found in pages 95, 96, 109, 165, 190.

3. Many of the remedies are antiphlogistic; and there is a certain stage, in almost every case of the disease, in which tonics do material injury.

4. The frequent buffiness of the blood, and that too sometimes of a peculiar kind, is not to be overlooked in this investigation; and it is worthy of much notice, that whilst the blood and the secreted serum are accused of being too watery, the urine, which commonly contains little or no albumen, is loaded with it in a great and unnatural proportion. This phænomenon could hardly be expected as the result of too thin a condition of the fluids, and a deficiency of coagulable matter; on the contrary, it is a very strong proof, if not

of its excess, at least of some newly-ac-
quired properties with regard to separation,
and of an altered texture.   I add as a
fact on which we cannot too often reflect,
that where the urine is most loaded, coagulates by the lowest heat, and most firmly,
the blood is likewise most buffy, and the
whole system bears the greatest marks of
inflammation.

The coagulable state of the urine, being
so intimately connected with the presence
of an extravasated and stagnated serum,
may be thought perhaps to be furnished
immediately from that source.   And it
was I suppose an observation of this sort
that induced Dr. Darwin to believe, as has
been already stated, that the serum passed
into the bladder by an inverted motion
of the lymphatic system.   Such a supposition receives no kind of support from
anatomy, and is even contradicted by the
valvular structure of those vessels.   But is

the other part of that most ingenious
author's suggestion, whose very conjectures
are the intuitive glances of a superior mind
into the secrets of nature, less open to
objection? Is it in short possible that,
according to the common course of the circulation, the dropsical accumulations may
supply the albumen in the urine?

It may be urged as a strong presumptive
evidence of the truth of this doctrine, that
the discharge alluded to is hardly ever
found but in dropsical habits; and there is
no reason whatever to deny, that even in
such habits a constant absorption is going
on, not indeed equal to the increased exhalation, yet still so far answering its purpose for many months together, that the
patient becomes rather emaciated than
much swelled. If the fluid has been so
vitiated, as to be wholly unfit for the
purposes of circulation, it remains that
nature should discharge it by some of the
emunctories. The kidneys, from the comparative simplicity of their secretion, are
probably the glands most suited to such
an office. They appear to be possessed of
a sort of elective power, capable of sepa-

rating from the blood whatever is hurtful to it. The urine is perpetually impregnated both in smell and colour with foreign materials. The examples of its containing even a purulent deposit, in consequence of sudden translations from abscesses in remote parts of the body, are too well authenticated to admit of doubt; and Dr. Heberden's authority may be quoted for this fact, not from a neglect of what former writers have asserted on the subject, but because no one will consider him to have been either credulous in belief, or inaccurate in observation. *

This doctrine seems plausible, but there are several very strong objections to it.

1st. It does not at all account for the presence of red blood in the urine, which occasionally renders this discharge a true hæmorrhage.

2d. The urine has been in some degree coagulable by heat, in a body not dropsical, where the cavity of the abdomen has been filled with pus.

3d. The same result has taken place,

* Heberden's Commentaries, page 472.

where no fluid of any sort has been accumulated to supply its materials. *

4th. This discharge has been observed to a considerable extent in hydrocephalus,

* This was very observable in a man in whom dissection proved the total absence of all dropsy. His symptoms were an imaginary syphilis, accompanied by an earnest desire to take mercury, from which I thought it probable that he had already taken too much of it; hypochondriasis; irritation of the urinary organs; a vomiting in the middle of the night of a black bile and indigested food, or of a very frothy matter ; stools of a similar nature, great difficulty of moving the bowels, excessive emaciation and despondency.

The whole disease was found to be seated in the stomach. Near the cardia was a cicatrized ulcer, in the inner membrane, of the size of a shilling; at the great end, and round the pylorus, there were extensive cicatrices of ulcers; and fleshy bands passed quite across that opening, acting as an almost complete valve to it. In one part where the stomach lay over the pancreas, its muscular substance had been destroyed entirely, and the pancreas was quite visible through the healed surface, or rather formed that surface itself. The substance of the pylorus was free from any scirrhosity. There was no open ulcer to be found in any part; all had healed, and in some places with rather exuberant granulations. The black fluid passed up on pressure from the duodenum. Every thing else was sound and in order.

T

where the collected fluid is both diluted and very small in quantity.

5th. It assumes its severest and most aggravated form, whilst all the other circumstances of the disease are increasing; *i. e.* at the moment when we should expect absorption to be the least active; and instantly decreases, when the relief which the patient experiences shows the accumulated matter to be passing off, or in other words the action of the absorbents to be carried on with increasing vigour.

6th. This supposition is still less capable of accounting for the almost total absence of albumen in the urine of common symptomatic dropsy, in which, however, we cannot doubt the absorption to be active, if not during the increase of the disease, at least during its cure.

These objections are very strong, nor do they admit of an answer in any part, but by acknowledging that great difference in the nature of dropsies, which it has been a principal object of this volume to point out, and by supposing that, where the serum is present in the urine, it has already been secreted into the affected cavities in an unusually disordered state. Some of the phænomena, however, are not explained even on this admission; particularly the presence of red blood in the urine, and of serum where the accumulation has been either purulent or none, and still further its rapid return to a natural state, the moment the removal of the swellings begins to take place. These facts render it probable, that the remarkable symptom above mentioned is not connected with any previous absorption of vitiated fluid, but with some cause more directly affecting the constitution. Either supposition involves considerations of great importance. If the coagulable part of the urine is supplied from the dropsical cavity, disease of that cavity is indicated, probably of the inflammatory kind, more than is essential to a mere dropsy; if some other parts of the system are in fault, the change thus indicated, though at present obscure, is undoubtedly of high importance, and demands particular correctives. The general phænomena of the disease seem to be best explained on the latter of these suppositions; but what the nature of this change may be, whether the blood is presented for secretion in a vitiated state, and in what manner vitiated, or the urinary organs themselves perform their office imperfectly, is at present not well ascertained. So far certainly we may be confident, that this sign can never have its proper weight, unless we view it in conjunction with the other symptoms, and as forming part of that great constitutional derangement, by which the organs of digestion and assimilation are impaired, the blood and its secretions vitiated, the cavities filled with fluid, their fine membranes injured, and even the complexion itself gradually marked with tokens of danger and decay, too decisive to be misunderstood. As a sign therefore of such a state of health, this symptom is invaluable; and to neglect or misinterpret it, will be to deprive ourselves of the strongest evidence which the disease can afford, and of the principal means of relieving it.

Suspicions of an inflammatory state in dropsy are not new ; and authors have long since mentioned, that the blood is buffy in some circumstances of that distemper.

Alexander Trallian and Paulus Ægineta recommend bleeding in anasarca.

Spon in his *novi Aphorismi* relates a case which was cured by twenty venæ-sections, after it had resisted hydragogues and diuretics.

Dr. Home in his Clinical Experiments states, that he succeeded by seven bleedings in seventeen days, and that the blood was inflamed.

Dr. Stock speaks with greater precision when he remarks, that the various species of hydropical affection are more frequently attended with a sthenic diathesis, than is generally apprehended ; that the arterial action is sometimes tense, but more frequently oppressed, and is found to increase in force and activity after the use of depleting remedies. He adds, that dropsy has been defined by some practical writers to be an inflammatory disease, accompanied by watery effusion. *

Dr. Grapengiesser, in his dissertation *de hydrope plethorico*, appears to treat this subject more fully than any other author, and in a very original manner. As the work, however, is not for sale in London, I speak only from the review which is given of it in Dr. Duncan's Medical Commentaries; to which Mr. Burns, in the course of some remarks on the same subject, has referred his reader. †

The author above alluded to considers the plethoric dropsy to occur much more commonly, than is suspected. He states it to come on suddenly in robust habits, slowly in weak ones, and to be attended by signs of peripneumony, with an inflamed blood. Much relief is experienced from large bleedings at the nose, and small repeated venæ-sections, and from neutral salts. Common diuretics and strong purges do harm. The former species, or sudden attack, he

* Stock's Medical Collections on Cold, p. 158.
† Burns on Diseases of the Heart.

has found readily curable by the anti-phlogistic treatment, the latter with great difficulty curable by any means, but certainly only by that treatment cautiously adopted.

Mr. Cruickshank's experiments, which ascertain that the urine in general dropsy differs from the natural in coagulating by heat, nitrous acid, and the corrosive sublimate, prove likewise that in inflammatory diseases, as peripneumony and acute rheumatism, a similar effect is produced by corrosive sublimate, and sometimes by nitrous acid.

Mr. Watts's case of diabetes, No. III. was certainly a dropsical one. The blood drawn was buffy, and a cure was obtained by repeated venæ-sections.

My own observations confirm and, I hope, illustrate these, and render it highly probable, that this inflammatory disposition prevails in those cases principally in which the urine is coagulable.

Buffiness of the blood has been considered by some practitioners as no very conclusive evidence of inflammation. I believe

however, that unless in the pregnant state
it very rarely indeed, if ever, occurs, but
as indicating and supporting some active
and morbid process ; and its presence in
pregnancy is rather a confirmation of this
opinion.   That state, though not diseased,
is greatly different from common health ;
and the system is very actively engaged
in the formation of new parts.   There
can be little doubt, from the uniform
harmony of nature and her doing nothing in vain, that this buffy condition
of the blood, with its power of remaining fluid for an unusual time, is the best
suited to such processes, and is intimately connected with them.   The disorders likewise of pregnancy are highly
inflammatory, and often require venæ-
section.   Still further, when on other occasions inflammation takes place, and
lymph is copiously deposited, as in acute
rheumatism, the blood becomes similarly
affected.

Whenever then such a process is suspected and blood is drawn, it will surely
be a great confirmation of those suspi-

cions, and an encouragement to the practitioner, if he finds it to possess those
qualities, which nature herself has chosen
when she forms new parts, and which so
frequently attend on a morbid extravasation of lymph.

CHAPTER XV.

THE SAME SUBJECT CONTINUED.

OF THE CURE.

SECTION I.

Blood–letting. —— Blisters.

STAHL remarks, that hæmorrhages are
cured by moderate depletion, but by the
use of astringents and tonics are converted
into dropsies; and our practice will be rational in dropsy itself, in proportion as we
keep the spirit of this observation in our
view. The loss of the serous part of the
blood, which so remarkably distinguishes
it, presents to us a symptom of a very debilitating kind; and our first consideration
of the subject might naturally enough en-

courage us to attempt its cure by those remedies which, from their effects on occasions not apparently dissimilar, are called astringents. If, however, the doctrine of Stahl is ever true in an actual inflammatory hæmorrhage, it is certainly most strictly so with regard to this flux of serum. Whoever endeavours to restrain it by bark, steel, and similar remedies, will inevitably see reason to repent that attempt, in an increased tension and fulness, a puffy countenance, a cough if there has been already none, and in worse cases, a true peripneumony. The very symptom for which he has prescribed will likewise be aggravated. Experience more than enough has convinced me of the truth and importance of this observation. Not indeed, that practitioners can be said generally to act in contradiction in it; for they have too much overlooked the appearance to which it relates, to have made its removal an object of their contemplation. But it is so common an error in practice to impute discharges to debility, and endeavour to check them by astringents, that it cannot be too much provided against.

The indications which they have usually followed in dropsies, are,

1st. To evacuate the accumulated fluid.

2d. To prevent a return of the accumulation by tonic remedies.

These arise obviously from the symptoms, as Sydenham observes, and are correct as far as they extend. But they are not sufficiently comprehensive for all cases, nor have a sufficient reference to some peculiar and striking circumstances of the hydropic diathesis, of which the watery accumulations form sometimes but a small part, and seldom deserve that exclusive attention which they receive. I allude especially to those signs of inflammation of the habit, which are not unfrequently present. That practitioner, I am confident, will treat the disorder most easily, most successfully, most suitably to the feelings of the patient, who keeps the probability of it in his view; and his attempts at cure must

perpetually prove abortive, unless in selecting his hydragogue medicines, he
prefers those which are likewise calculated to reduce inflammation. But it
may be necessary to go beyond this,
and to pursue a treatment more directly antiphlogistic. There are likewise cases, in which the indication to
evacuate the water can have little place,
since hardly any is collected, but in
which the system suffers more severely and
under a more intense inflammation, than
is usual in very extensive dropsies. Here
the correction of that error in the habit
must uniformly precede every attempt to
strengthen it.

The most powerful of these antiphlogistic agents is venæ-section, a remedy
which no one would wish to employ in
any disease without necessity, and particularly revolting to the general opinion in
œdematous swellings. I have, however,
directed it in several such instances, and
never had reason to regret its use. The
state of the blood, and the relief that followed, have usually confirmed the propriety

12

of the operation.　　It is most obviously
called for by the accession of pneumonia;
I believe likewise, that the disease occasionally falls on the abdomen in such a
manner, as equally to require it; and that
it is likely to be of particular service after
mercurial courses, where the urine is
greatly increased in quantity, and in the
inflammatory anasarca.　It is indeed sometimes the only evacuation which can be directed for cachectic patients, their stomach
rejecting both laxatives and diuretics;
whilst the ease with which they undergo
this operation, as well as the relief they
experience from it, are truly surprising.
A correct guide to it may be found in the
firmness, copiousness, and early appearance of coagulum in the urine; its limits,
in the improvement of that discharge, the
state of the blood, and the relief of the
other symptoms.

Imperfectly, however, as this subject has
hitherto been considered, it will be pru-
dent at first to prescribe it with caution
as to quantity, and under those circumstances in which the nature of the cause

and of the signs cannot mislead us. Certainly it is not to be viewed with that extreme suspicion, which is sometimes entertained against all weakening remedies in chronic ailments; and there are periods of the disorder, in which no other operation can preserve life.

When internal inflammation is suspected, blisters near the affected part are very serviceable; if applied to the extremities, in order to evacuate the dropsical fluid, though they often fulfil that temporary object, they produce great danger of sloughing ulcers, and now and then a troublesome irritation in the course of the lymphatics.

SECTION II.

Purgatives; elaterium, gamboge, jalap, &c.
tartrate and supertartrate of pot-ash; and
tartarized soda. — Antimonials.

THE other remedies against inflammation
are fortunately the same as have been
usually prescribed for the purpose of evacuating the accumulated fluid.

This indication is fulfilled principally by
certain purgatives and diuretics.

It has been, more perhaps than it is at
present, the custom to employ drastic purgatives, scammony, gamboge, elaterium,
jalap, the expressed juice of the root of the
common fleur-de-luce, hellebore, &c.; and
they undoubtedly have the power of evacuating large quantities of watery fluid, as
their name, hydragogue, implies. The objections to their use are, the temporary
heat and fever which they are apt to excite,

in allusion to which, Pliny says of the black hellebore, *quod medetur hydropicis citra febrim*; the uncertainty and distress of their operation in patients difficult to be purged; the rapid re-accumulation of the water; and the necessity which exists on that account for their almost daily repetition, till the swellings are entirely removed.

It is likewise obvious that, if the complaint is not carried off by these means, it must be aggravated by them; and an increased debility will follow, paticularly of the digestive organs. Some authors speak of a colliquative force which they possess, and of their dissolving the blood; expressions however incorrect in theory, yet intelligible in a practical view. And Hoffman asserts that he has seen them in an ascites produce an inflammation of the bowels, followed speedily by sphacelus.

Notwithstanding these grounds for alarm, yet where the habit is indolent and free from gout, and the dropsy extensive, without fever or local determination, they are, generally speaking, safe, and productive of a considerable effect. It is, however,

U

to such cases, certainly the most curable
form of the disease by other means, that
they are chiefly applicable.   In the cachexy, in which the stomach and intestines are very weak, they do such injury,
as to be wholly inadmissible; and agreeably to that excellent aphorism of Bag-
livi, *in morbis pectoris ad vias urinæ du-
cendum*, I have not seen them render any
service in the hydrothorax.   On the
other hand, they have produced in some
instances this partial effect, that whilst
they have relieved the cellular membrane,
they have left the chest oppressed, the
urine inflamed and loaded with serum,
and the whole system incapable of bearing any tonic remedies.   Indiscriminately
employed therefore, they must be attended with much hazard; and as a general plan of treatment, I have observed
them greatly fail, even in hands otherwise skilful.   Altogether their use is much
less extended since the introduction of
digitalis, and of the proper mode of
exhibiting crystals of tartar; and without
much injury to the practice of physic, may
perhaps be safely superseded by these.

If active purging is determined on, elaterium may be given in the dose of two or three grains, or gamboge as recommended in the later practice of Dr. Cullen, three grains repeated every three or four hours, till it has a considerable effect; or from twenty to thirty grains of jalap, with double that quantity of crystals of tartar. A combination of mild with drastic purgatives has been particularly recommended in persons difficult to be purged, whom strong medicines alone greatly ruffle and disturb. Formulæ of this kind are well known; but I avoid entering into the detail of these, or indeed any formulæ, because it would be to load the work with an useless repetition of what others have said, and what the persons, for whom I write, know; and my object at present is rather a more precise application of remedies, than any novel combination of them.

Drastic purgatives have sometimes been united with chalybeates, as in the celebrated electuary of Dovar, which is a combination of scammony, chalybs cum sulphure ppt., and crude antimony; and

u 2

which was likewise adopted by Dr. Hugh
Smith. *   The dose prescribed by him is
from fifteen to thirty grains of the first of
these ; and twelve grains each of the two
others.   I have known the sulphate of
iron substituted for the chalybs cum sulphure.   This formula has undoubtedly
performed many cures ; and there is so
much debility in the disease, that the
addition of tonics to purgatives, never
indifferent, is particularly desirable here,
whenever it can be made with safety.

In proportion as the complaint assumes
an inflammatory aspect, the saline purgatives are undoubtedly more required ;
they are, in the truest sense of the word,
aperient, diuretic as well as laxative, and
promoting all the excretions.   Whilst they
unload, they cool, without leaving that
extreme debility of the intestines, so much
to be dreaded from hydragogues ; and
the constitution is rendered by their use
daily more and more fit for the exhibition
of tonics.

There can, I think, be no hesitation in

* Smith's Formulæ, p. 20.

preferring those salts into the composition of which the tartaric acid enters ; as the tartrate of pot-ash, the supertartrate of pot-ash or crystals of tartar, and the tartarized soda.

If from the circumstances of the case a decidedly laxative effect is required, the first or the last of these may be usefully combined in the quantity of half an ounce, with infusion, and tincture, of senna, or tincture of jalap.

But there is likewise something very advantageous in the influence which saline remedies exert, by being given in such a form as to enter the circulation, and of themselves to open the secretions, which are undoubtedly deficient in dropsy; those from the skin, the kidneys, and the bowels, obviously so. With this intention, the supertartrate of pot-ash is usually selected, and is given from half an ounce to an ounce daily, diluted with water only, or with such additions as are necessary to render it agreeable to the stomach. The mildness of this remedy, the length of time during which it can be continued in a smaller dose as a dietetic, the solvent power which it seems to exert over the cause of the distemper, place it in the very first rank. How much more satisfactory and more likely to be permanent is such a cure, than that which tears to pieces, whilst it unloads? It approaches to the cure by diet, which undoubtedly is the most desirable of all, and imitates most nearly the operations of nature. A scanty urine, loaded with a lateritious sediment and with serum, is an indication for the use of this as well as other saline remedies. It is contra-indicated by a pale watery condition of that discharge, in which likewise there is generally a predominant acid, and by a certain appearance of feebleness in the kidneys. Often, I believe, it unloads the urine entirely. I have known it do so partially only; but with such effect, that tonics easily perform the rest.

Antimonial remedies are well calculated to overcome a phlogistic state, and on the other hand, wherever they render benefit, it seems probable that the disease has possessed that character. The encomiums passed on their use in dropsy, by

Sydenham, are not without considerable foundation. His expressions are very strong, when he says, that antimonial emetics do not seem merely to evacuate the stomach, but to open some passages from the cavity of the abdomen into the intestinal canal. * Without, however, employing this mineral so freely and largely as that great author did, much benefit may be derived by joining it in a smaller doze, ¼ gr. of tartarized antimony, or in a fluid form one drachm of the liquor

---

* These expressions of Sydenham approach so nearly to the opinions entertained by Dr. Darwin, respecting some secret communication between cavities not apparently communicating with each other but by the route of the circulation, that I will subjoin his own words.

" Necesse est omnino, ut cum tanta fuerit agitatio
" concussioque tam ventriculi quam viscerum, à tam
" insigni aquarum corrivatione quasi circumseptorum,
" earundem evacuatio per ductus, communi naturæ
" lege haud satis patentes, conatum ita vehementem in-
" sequatur. Quod vero dentur ejusmodi cœci meatus,
" per quos aquæ ex abdominis cavitate ad intestina
" transferantur, de facto liquet; cum quotidié observe-
" mus Hydragoga tantam aquarum in abdomine in-
" clusarum vim per recessum educere, perinde ac si
" primitus in ipsis intestinis continerentur."—Sydenham.
Opera Universa, p. 489.

u 4

antimonii tartarizati, with laxatives. It
greatly promotes their operation, and
suits the intention with which they are
given, and corrects any of their heating
qualities.

Those who expect to derive most benefit
from purging, lay it down as an indispen-
sable rule, that it should be repeated as
frequently as the strength of the patient
can possibly bear, almost daily, or at the
least two or three times a week, till the
water is removed. I suppose there is
much propriety in this direction, and that
on any other plan the swellings return
rapidly; because we see it adopted with
regard to the mildest laxatives, the soluble tartar, cream of tartar, &c. as well
as the strongest; and probably in this
respect the former have a great advantage over the latter, that they can be
persisted in daily without detriment to the
patient.

SECTION III.

Diuretics; Squills; Oil of Turpentine: Can-
tharides; Sulphate of Copper; Acetate of
Pot-ash, &c.; Tobacco; Digitalis; Infu-
sion of Broom-tops, &c.—— Of Tincture of.
Opium. —— Tapping. —— Scarifications.

THE urine is so generally affected in dropsical swellings, as very naturally to suggest
the use of diuretics. Medicines of this class,
however, are allowed by the best authors to
be uncertain in their effect; nor is it at all
reasonable to expect, that the same remedy
should be indiscriminately serviceable in
such very different conditions of the urinary
secretion as have been above described.

I have stated, from an experience which
I trust cannot mislead, that squill is much
to be depended on, where, with an oppression of the chest, the urine is scanty, high-
coloured, full of sediment, and without
serum. Its use, however, is not limited to

this state. I have sometimes seen it render service, where the urine is partially coagulable. But in proportion as that symptom becomes more marked by its extreme constitutional characters, inflammation, and a weakness of the digestive organs, it fails in its effect, or is even injurious. Particularly the debility and loss of appetite that result from it are often rapid and excessive. I have seldom had so much reason to regret the use of medicine, as of squill in these circumstances ; and where they are present, even the affection of the chest, so greatly relieved by it at other times, does not justify its exhibition.

It is in the inflammatory dropsy particularly, that those authors who at all notice its existence, assert the common diuretics to be improper. This assertion must be accepted with some limitations, and with a due consideration of their general properties. Those diuretics which possess a stimulating power, as the oil of turpentine and the other natural balsams, and the cantharides, or an astringent and tonic one, as the preparations of copper, are without doubt wholly unsuitable to such a state. Yet some

15

authors have spoken much in their praise in dropsy. The powder of cantharides, from ¼ gr. to one or two grains, has been recommended in extreme cases by Lieutaud, and asserted by him to form the basis of an active empirical remedy. The preparations of copper have been highly extolled by Boerhaave, Dr. Wright, and others. That these remedies have no specific power in correcting that remarkable condition of the urine so often mentioned, I have ascertained by repeated experiments; I have even thought that the tincture of cantharides has increased this tendency to coagulation. The authority, however, of such physicians leaves me in no doubt, that this treatment may render benefit under some circumstances of the disease; what they are, we can at present only conjecture, from the obvious and known qualities of the remedies themselves.

In proportion as stimulating diuretics are improper, we naturally turn to those, which cool and attenuate, or which diminish inflammatory action. Such are;

1st. The saline remedies already mentioned, under the head of laxatives, parti-

cularly the crystals of tartar. One of the
neutral salts, the acetate of pot-ash, has so
high a character in this respect, that it has
even received the distinguishing name,
among the old writers of sal diureticus,
with what justice, I can hardly determine.
Dr. Heberden thinks that the Rochelle
salt and the soluble tartar have an equal
claim to it.

With the pot-ash I have not succeeded.
Nor is there any reasonable expectation,
that where the crystals of tartar are advisable, the alkali can be beneficial; perhaps; however, it may be well suited to
those circumstances of the disease, in which
the urine is pale, and not scanty, and remains long free from putrefraction.

2d. Tobacco. — Dr. Fowler's reports leave
no doubt of its efficacy; and its very en-
feebling influence on the constitution leaves
as little, that the disease which it over-
comes must be at least combined with some
stricture or inflammation. I speak, however, from no particular experience of its
efficacy.

3d. Digitalis. — This plant has certainly
made a great addition of late years to our

means of cure. For although before the time of Dr. Withering's publication on that subject it had been employed very frequently, both in this and other countries, as a domestic drug, yet its exhibition was regulated by no sort of principle or distinction ; and accuracy, as to dose, was wholly out of the question. Even lately, the common people of this neighbourhood have been in the habit of using very strong and copious infusions of it, made by throwing boiling water on the leaves, stem, and root, without any measure or weight. The results have been some unexpected recoveries much talked of, and more failures, which tell no tales. Dr. Withering by showing its safety as well as its efficacy, and by greatly diminishing the dose, has taken the only means of rendering it applicable to common use. I have endeavoured to add something to those signs which should direct its exhibition.

Digitalis very generally cures dropsy after scarlatina, when attended by coagulable urine, and sometimes even the hydrocephalus from that cause. It is particularly certain in its action, where the urine is likewise turbid and deposits a bloody sediment. Should it be found uniformly to fail, as it has done in my hands, where an opposite condition of that discharge prevails, that very exception will throw great light both on the nature of this symptom and of the remedy.

It is likewise very advantageously employed in this disease, when arising from other causes, provided the habit be not yet entirely depraved nor the substance of the viscera affected; and a positive inflammation of the blood has at least formed no impediment to its success. Can we think that it is any thing but an encouragement? But many of all these are cases in which other means of relief, as occasional venæ-section, mild purging, saline diuretics, may be resorted to with advantage. It is in circumstances nearly thought desperate by other treatment, in the hydrothorax in which even squills fail, that digitalis exerts a power truly astonishing. In many such instances, it acts both speedily and in small doses, and gives a relief wholly unlooked for. It is not too much to say, that lives are prolonged for many years by the discreet management of this remedy alone; and that by the rash mixture with it of other diuretics, and of mercurial deobstruents, the greatest risk is incurred of entirely changing the whole result.

In proportion as visceral disease prevails, less certainly is to be expected from this or any other diuretic; but in many mixed cases, and where the accumulations are provoked by intemperance, it repeatedly relieves.

When the organs of digestion fail, and there is a constant diarrhœa or sickness, and the bad habit of the body is more remarkable than the extent or seat of the dropsy, it has appeared to be rather injurious, by causing a still further debility of the stomach. In one instance of this kind, however, which was very unpromising, after bleeding, digitalis combined with opium succeeded. * An open ulcer of the lungs is likewise a great objection to it; and it never performs a cure, whilst it purges.

Without any particular reference to the other symptoms, and even where the patient

* Pages 147 and 148.

has not been visited, the state of the urine itself furnishes an important indication on this subject.   If besides partially coagulating by heat, it is rather scanty, and not deficient in colour, foul when made and containing some red blood, or becoming turbid when cold and depositing a branny or lateritious sediment, I expect much from the employment of digitalis.   If, on the contrary, the urinary secretion, however loaded with serum, is pale and crude, much more if copious, the service derived from it will be very partial, and the dose must be small ; and it will be well if it does no injury.   I must confess further, that even where the signs, which I have thought favourable for its use, were combined, the constitution of the patient was such, as to render its continuance impossible, in consequence of a pain over one eye ; and this on repeated trials, in very small doses.   And it is worthy of notice, that in the patient to whom I particularly allude, some blood drawn at the commencement of this plan was not inflamed.

There are some considerations not to be overlooked in selecting the preparations of

this drug; but they are of less importance
than its dose, and the length of time during which it should be continued. The
dried leaf is undoubtedly the strongest of
these preparations, and would generally
be entitled to a preference, if it were not
that in an application of such activity,
and where small errors may be very serious, we rather wish to be possessed of the
means of accurately measuring it, than
giving it in a very concentrated shape.
On this account a solution is to be preferred, independently of the superior facility of absorption which it may possibly
furnish; and as this plant gives out its
virtues to boiling water, there seems no reasonable objection of any kind to the infusion. On the other hand, there are many
advantages in varying the mode of exhibition as little as possible; for which reason
I have thought it right to adhere in this
work to the proportions directed by the
L. P. and copied with very little variation
from Dr. Withering; one drachm of the
dried leaves to half a pint of boiling water,
to which is added, after straining, half an
ounce of spirit of cinnamon; although the

x

dose is often necessarily so small, as to
make it convenient in extemporaneous
prescription to direct an infusion of less
strength.   Our first object, undoubtedly,
should be to choose such doses of it, as
will cure ;   our second, carefully to avoid
such as may act with violence or offence.
For it is not always enough to stop its use,
when this bad effect has taken place.   A
disgust so excited is generally very permanent, and not merely a disgust, but sometimes a total inability of the stomach to
admit the offending substance.   Persons
who have once suffered in this way, frequently cannot, by any persuasion or even
determination of the mind, be prevailed on
to risk a repetition ; a state very much to
be avoided, in a disease so liable to re-
lapses, and with such limited means of
relief.

Considering therefore, that two ounces
of the infusion, or an infusion of fifteen
grains, is the largest quantity that should
be given in twenty-four hours, and that
from three to four drachms is the smallest
from which an adult, under common circumstances, can expect relief ; I should

recommend, that in proportion as the
habit is sound, the swellings extensive,
·and the urine loaded, from an ounce to an
ounce and half should be given in the day,
divided into two or three doses, and to
be augmented to the extreme quantity, if
required; and that where the age is advanced, the stomach very feeble, the accumulation seated principally in the chest,
the viscera suspected, the urine but slightly
coagulating and perhaps crude, we should
commence with the smallest of these quan-
.tities; and it will be much more easy to
increase the dose, than it will have been
safe to produce the necessity for diminishing
it. In children, as after scarlatina, it should
be of course proportioned to the age; less
than a drachm will often be sufficient; and
it is of great importance to recollect, that
as there is no circumstance in which constitutions vary more than in their suscepti-
bility to the bad effects of digitalis, we can
hardly err by excessive caution.

In the feeble habits which this remedy
peculiarly assists, opium often forms an
adjunct of some consequence, and may
be given combined with it in small doses,

particularly to prevent purging, or as a full anodyne at night, which will be found serviceable in that restlessness, spasmodic dyspnœa, and nightly micturition, that sometimes accompany the hydrothorax. I have seen the diuretic action both of squills and digitalis greatly assisted by opium. Generally speaking, no other addition will be required, except the watery vehicle which is necessary to put it into a convenient form, and perhaps in weak stomachs, some spirit or tincture, at the choice of the prescriber. If laxatives are wanted, they should be of the mildest kind, never such as to produce diarrhœa, or carry the medicine downwards ; and on this account they had better perhaps not be exhibited together, unless where the occasion is very urgent.

This treatment will, if justly directed, be followed in a few days by some relief of the symptoms ; and the state of the urine will be generally amongst the first and most convincing signs of this. It not only becomes apparently more diluted, but on examination by heat daily precipitates less. Can there be a more satisfactory evidence of the benefit of the remedy ; and that the cause of the disease is reached by it, as far at least as the watery accumulations are concerned? Whenever it removes the swellings without this favourable change, I have not seen any permanent advantage from it, or from any thing else; but the patient usually dies emaciated, or convulsed and tympanitic.

Sometimes during an unguarded continuance of digitalis, a coagulum has reappeared in the urine, but so loose, and attended by so many other signs of feebleness that I have been able to subdue it by immediately having recourse to the Peruvian bark.

Notwithstanding our utmost caution, symptoms may come on, certainly not necessary to the beneficial action of the remedy, but rather obstructing it, and which should be the signal for its immediate discontinuance. These are, retardation of the pulse, palpitations, faintness, sickness, and purging. There is likewise a membranous tensive pain of the head, sometimes over one eye, with a sort of disturbance of the brain, which occasionally atends an overdose, before any other bad signs have ap-

x 3

peared, but which has not been noticed as it ought to be by any writer. If neglected, it is followed by convulsions. It comes on in persons who bear the medicine very badly, and in small doses only; and who are never much relieved by it. If even the diuretic effects are considerable, its use should be suspended, or at least the quantity much lessened; since the same dose, which was barely sufficient for breaking down the obstruction to that secretion, of whatever kind it was, proves too powerful when that obstruction is removed, and the tone of the system already lowered. This appears plausible in theory, it is certainly experimentally true; and it is the more important to enforce it, since it is natural for patients, and is indeed the custom of some practitioners, to push the remedy, whenever it begins to operate favourably, and as they could wish. Nothing can be more pregnant with mischief than such a practice.

Not so much to increase this catalogue of bad effects, as to guard against them, I add from the observation of more than one very experienced practitioner, that sudden death occurs in an unusual proportion, where digitalis has been exhibited in large doses ; and this, either before the signs above enumerated have appeared, or before they have been noticed. It will not be thought superfluous to repeat, what constant experience more and more impresses on my mind, that the avoiding what are called excessive doses, is but a small part of the caution with which it should be exhibited, and that there are cases in which very minute quantities of it are positively injurious, I might almost say, poisonous. This state I have usually found designated by a remarkable paleness and want of feverish sediment in the urine ; on the other hand the most striking and complete examples of its success have been preceded by some appearance of foulness and red blood, as well as serum, in that discharge, similar to the character observed after scarlatina.

The antidotes against the poisonous effects of digitalis were stated in the former editions of this work to be,——blisters to the pit of the stomach ; from thirty to forty drops of tincture of opium in warm brandy and water; and if that cannot be retained, or the patient is too insensible to swallow, an opiate injection. These recommendations were given, partly on the authority of Dr. Withering, partly from some circumstances that had occurred to myself. But the observations of other practitioners have since made me doubt their propriety, particularly where the head is much affected; and, I trust, I shall never have experience enough on this subject in my own practice, to enable me to speak decidedly.

The least safe mode of exhibiting it, and the most likely to be followed by these bad consequences, is its repetition in full doses at short intervals, as every two or three hours, till it produces some sensible effect. This has been strongly objected to by Dr. Withering; because many hours often elapse before the effects of the former doses are visible, and a dangerous accumulation may take place, although none of the signals for forbearance have appeared. This practice was very common at first, it has not even yet wholly fallen into disuse. And it is perhaps possible that a situation of extreme urgency may justify it; but I conceive it to be much too hazardous for common practice, and wholly inapplicable to the ordinary circumstances of the disorder.

Dr. Withering was in the latter part of his practice disposed to believe, that smaller quantities than he had been in the habit of prescribing, viz. about two or three grains of the powder daily, remove the disorder gradually, with no other than mild diuretic effects, and without any interruption to their use, till the cure is completed. Even these doses, however, are not free from the possibility of injury, not fit to be continued without the watchful care of the medical attendant. The most experienced practitioner on this subject, I ever knew, has often told me, that he never again would order digitalis in dropsy, unless he had the means of visiting his patient daily. In phthisis pulmonalis, where there is less danger of a sudden collapse, trusting it to patients themselves is not without hazard, and I am persuaded has sometimes been attended with effects more immediately fatal than the disease itself. Even during the mild diuretic effect to which Dr. Withering alludes, it should be remembered, that the quality of the discharge is also gradually corrected; a less violent impression on the system is therefore daily called for, and less can be endured; and an easy diminution of the dose will be safe and advisable, if not necessary.

One considerable source of inaccuracy certainly arises from the various forms in which this medicine is prescribed, of infusion, tincture, and powder, (for the decoction may be neglected,) and the extreme difficulty of making a just calculation of the relative strength of these. It is a point that can only be determined by the nicest experiments on the sick; and we well know how many circumstances may occur to falsify such results. It has always appeared to me that the activity of the infusion prescribed by Dr. Withering is greater in comparison with the powder, than has been generally allowed; and he is not wholly consistent with himself in this particular.

Page 181. He considers, the dose of the powder to be from one grain to three grains twice a day in adults, and four grains a day to be sufficient in the reduced state in which physicians generally find dropsical patients.

Page 182. He says, that one ounce of the infusion twice a day is a medium dose for an adult; that in urgent cases it may be repeated every eight hours, and that in many instances half an ounce is sufficient. It appears then that he thought one ounce of the infusion, or an infusion of between seven and eight grains, to be equivalent to two grains of the powder.

A few lines after he adds, that thirty grains of the powder, or eight ounces of the infusion, may generally be taken before nausea commences, which makes one ounce of the infusion equal to three grains and three quarters of the powder. I believe that the latter of these is the more correct estimate; and that an ounce of the infusion, instead of being a medium is a very large dose, and approaches to four grains of the powder. I speak, however, of this latter, from a knowledge comparatively inaccurate; because I have, wherever it was possible, preferred the infusion, for the reasons before assigned. If there are decided objections to a liquid form, the powder may certainly be given made into pills, with soap, &c.

The saturated tincture has advantages over even the infusion in the extreme convenience of form, and its being always ready for use; but I must confess myself to entertain doubts, whether it possesses diuretic powers in an equal degree. Thirty drops, every eight hours, are the greatest quantity that can be exhibited with safety; and I have cured several adults by less than that quantity during the whole day.

If for preparing the infusion the fresh leaves are obtained more readily, an allowance must be made for the great loss of weight which they would have sustained by drying, as Dr. Maclean says, from 3-4ths to 4-5ths of the whole*, without a corresponding diminution of strength, so that the quantity of the herb used must be greater in about that proportion.

Accuracy in collecting and preserving this plant is of the utmost consequence. It possesses at all times considerable virtues, as its smell and taste indicate. But for the

* Medical and Physical Journal, vol. ii. page 122.

greater uniformity of strength, it should be gathered when beginning to flower, of course in the second year of its growth; care being taken to remove all the damaged leaves. It should be dried entire in a moderate heat, near the fire, or in the sunshine; and when sufficiently dried, the leaves should be set apart for use separating from them the leaf-stalk, and mid-rib. Particular caution is necessary in keeping them free from the access of air and moisture, but especially the latter. Too much attention cannot be paid to this circumstance. If the entire plant be permitted to remain in the open air for some months, especially where any dampness can affect it, it becomes totally inert, retaining indeed a bitter quality, but losing that faint poisonous effluvia with which its medical efficacy seems connected. The same deterioration happens from keeping the coarse powder in paper, or in a bottle which is often opened for use. I attribute it not less to such inattention than to its indiscriminate application, that practitioners entertain very unsettled notions of its effects, and frequently complain of its uncertain

action.   If we employ an infusion, and
that of an uniform strength, made from
the leaves carefully dried and kept, and
ascertain the exact character of the urinary
discharge before we do employ it, the obscurity, which has hitherto been complained
of, will not, I trust, long remain.

Dr. Maclean, in his able work on hydrothorax, has made some valuable remarks on
the action of digitalis.   His opinion coin-
cides entirely with that of Dr. Withering,
respecting the constitutions that admit of
most relief from it.   They both agree, that
it acts more favourably on a weak and lax
fibre, where the œdematous limbs readily
pit on pressure, and the complexion is pale
and transparent, less so in men of great natural strength, a chorded pulse, florid complexion, and hard skin.

These observations seem at first sight to
contradict the remarks contained in this
volume.   Upon further consideration, however, I think they may without difficulty be
reconciled with each other ; and the authority of such respectable practical writers is
too considerable, not to make me very desirous of enlisting it, if possible, in my favour.

The robust constitutions then, which they consider to resist the digitalis, appear to be the same as are subject to the dropsy described in Chapter IV., and in which I have observed calomel and squill to render the most service. On the other hand, the signs, which in their opinion indicate its employment, characterize the strictly dropsical habit, and are certainly, as they most truly assert, attendant on great feebleness of body, either natural or acquired. They have omitted further to notice, that in these cases the inflammatory state, long talked of in dropsy, is often superadded; and it appears probable that the success of digitalis may in a great measure depend on its power of relieving that very dangerous and obscure combination.

Dr. Withering certainly gives no countenance to that opinion, but on the contrary proposes reducing the inflammatory diathesis by other means, venæ-section, crystals of tartar, and even squills, previous to its exhibition. This fanciful scheme he confesses has only partially succeeded in his hands; then only, I

should imagine, when venæ-section has
been employed; for digitalis is second
in activity to no other remedy, and in
many cases of chronic inflammation not
even to that.   On this account some practitioners are averse to its use in dropsy,
and would justly be so, if dropsy were
as they believe a mere feebleness and inactivity of the parts concerned.   But it
is often far otherwise, and the antiphlogistic powers of the remedy would of
themselves lead us to suspect some inflammation in the disease.   In the phthisical cough, which has sometimes been
remarkably checked by the judicious management of digitalis, it is less easy to
entertain any doubts of this kind.   There
every thing plainly indicates an inflamed,
though delicate, habit.   Venæ-section is
often necessary; a light diet and mild
aperients render some service; and digitalis, by a more penetrating influence
than any of these, corrects the excessive
action of the arterial system.   This extraordinary controul, which it exercises
over the heart and arteries, can be indifferent in no disorder; and it is not un-

reasonable to suppose by analogy, even if the symptoms themselves did not often afford powerful arguments, that the great benefits which result from it in the dropsical habit, are neither in contradiction to its depressing powers, nor even independent of them ; but that there has been in the persons so relieved, some lurking inflammation, or stricture, and perhaps an altered texture of the blood, which digitalis only has been able to reach and break down.

So favourable a removal of the obstructing cause will naturally be followed by a restoration of all the secretions, but particularly that of the kidneys ; and the load of superfluous fluid, with which the vessels become inundated, must be thrown off by that gland principally. We know nothing of the specific power of digitalis in increasing the urinary discharge, nor is it rendered probable by its effect in other states of the body ; but it would be rash to determine that it is not, most strictly speaking, diuretic in this disorder, because it is not so in others.

Y

It may not perhaps be wholly unimportant to mention, that it strikes a dark colour with the solution of green vitriol. This property does not seem immediately connected with its action on the kidneys, but is certainly common to it with some other medicines esteemed diuretic, as the broom and the expressed juice of artichoke *; and with others that advantageously alter the quality, if not the quantity, of the urine, as the uva ursi.

Of the exact circumstances to which these minor diuretics are applicable, I cannot precisely speak ; but I have known them to be wholly unequal to some severe cases of the disorder.

Occasionally the tincture of opium, given to relieve pain or diarrhoea, has had a very beneficial effect on the other symptoms.

Dr. Willis states, that in a dropsical patient, who took large doses of laudanum to

* Bohea tea has likewise been said, when chewed in large quantities, to cure dropsy.

I 2

relieve pain after a syphilis badly cured, the dropsy, probably mercurial, was entirely carried off by the same means. *

Dr. Mead records an instance somewhat similar. †

Dr. Heberden says that he has known an anasarca sometimes cured by opiates at night, probably, as he adds, by the sweat they occasioned. ‡

Dr. Home proposes as a question, *Quare opiata urinæ profluvium adaugent et morbum sæpe tollunt ?* §

In this volume, p. 146 to 148, a case is mentioned, in which a very free use of opium, combined with a very small quantity of digitalis, performed a cure ; which had the most share in it, is difficult to say.

Opiates then, and in large doses, are worthy the attention of the practitioner in this disease.   But whether they benefit by their power of allaying irritation, or by par-

* Willis, Pharmaceut. Ration. part i. sect. vii. cap. i.

† Mead, Monita et Precepta Medica, cap. viii.

‡ Heberden's Commentaries, page 224.

§ Home, Principia Medicinæ, lib. iii. part i. sect. iii.

ticularly determining to the surface, is not ascertained. The combination of other sudorifics with this has been recommended in anasarca. I can say nothing of it from my own experience.

Another mode of carrying off the accumulated fluid is by scarifications of the lower extremities, and tapping in the ascites. That these operations have a great influence, not only on the parts which they evacuate, but on the constitution at large, is shown by the favourable change in the urine already noticed. But their benefit is by no means permanent, unless we have an opportunity of assisting them by other remedies to be hereafter mentioned. And scarifications in particular are rarely advisable on account of the sloughing ulcers which they are disposed to produce in the wounded part. Are issues and setons in a less depending situation likely to answer better?

SECTION IV.

Of Diet.

THE proper regulation of the diet in dropsy is very important, both as it relates generally to the nourishment of the body, and to the correcting of any particular acrimony that may be present. The dulness of the dropsical habit, and the nature of many of its remote causes, appear to demand a generous and stimulant diet, whilst the actual existence of inflammation places limits to this indulgence; and no sober person will think of urging the use of much wine and heavy food, where the membranes are positively inflamed, or the circulation obstructed. On the other hand, in strong constitutions, dropsies have been removed, and their return prevented, during a total abstinence from fermented liquors. The more common error proba-

Y 3

bly has been that of too cordial and stimulant a plan.

Fruits are carefully to be avoided by those
who suffer from a copious discharge of pale
urine ; and the soda water gives to this
symptom great relief.

The feelings of the patient are to be consulted as much as possible, particularly
with regard to dilution. Thirst is always a
sign of heat or acrimony, and is rarely not
to be gratified ; and I imagine, that the
instances of recovery under such an indulgence are beyond any comparison more
frequent than when a dry diet is attempted,
a regimen so barbarous and irrational, that
it is next to impossible to adhere to it.

In correcting the cause of this disease,
diet and medicinal articles of the most simple kind may probably be made great auxi-
liaries. The cure of scurvy, undoubtedly
a disease of the fluids, and so nearly allied to dropsy, that some cases may with
equal propriety receive either appellation,
gives great room for such a hope. And is
the history of dropsy itself less encourag-
ing in this respect ; when we recollect the
extreme characters of alkalescence and

acidity, which the urine sometimes indicates in it? These conditions, wholly incurable, as they have ever been found, by strong remedies directed to the solids and the nerves, may perhaps yield with an unexpected facility to their appropriate correctives, before mechanical injury of the nobler parts has succeeded to a general vitiation of the habit.

Hoffman informs us, that in dropsies amongst the lower orders, thought to be connected with a scorbutic taint, he has succeeded better with the antiscorbutic herbs, the horse-radish root, the juice of scurvy-grass, water-cress, and garden-cresses, and the decoction of the red beet, than with the most approved hydropic remedies; and that in such instances a very striking diuretic effect has followed their employment. * There are many similar examples which must suggest themselves to the recollection of every practitioner, where a recovery has been effected by alterations of diet not apparently great, and even sometimes accidental, as by the use of punch, light wines, &c.

* Hoffmanni Opera, tom. iii. page 233.

The question proposed by Dr. Home in his Principia, *Quare acida juvant?* implies the reality of the fact; and a just answer to this question would of itself solve many of our difficulties. *

My friend, Mr. Johnson, a surgeon of this city, and a practitioner of very accurate observation, informs me, that he was witness to a striking solution of the disease on board the Asia East-Indiaman, off Canton. Towards the conclusion of the voyage, the sailors had been attacked with dropsical symptoms, coming on very suddenly, and without those signs which are thought strictly to characterize scurvy, sponginess of the gums, and petechiæ. This disorder was attributed, no doubt with great reason, to the use of damaged rice, upon which, circumstances, not necessary to detail, had reduced them in a great measure to subsist. On their arrival in port, the principal improvement in their diet was well-fermented bread, which operated as a very active diuretic within twenty-four hours after they had begun its use; and no doubt

* Principia Medicinæ, de Hydrope.

remained in the minds of any of the sick, what it was that performed the cure. Those who preferred the native vegetable acids did not obtain the same immediate benefit. *

This is an example of a remarkable diuretic effect produced by an article of diet apparently very simple, but happily chosen. It is not, however, to the literal adoption of such a practice, but to the principle of it, that I wish to direct the attention of the reader, and to that facility of cure which results in scorbutic dropsies from an appropriate chemical corrective. How far this principle may be extended to common cases, in which there has been no extraor-

* In a collection of papers on the Diseases of Lascars in long voyages, published by Dr. Hunter, Calcutta, similar symptoms are described, certainly very nearly resembling the sea-scurvy, but marked perhaps by less of a putrid acrimony. It is, indeed, reasonable to suppose, that various depravations of food should produce disorders differing from each other in some respects, although they have a general character of resemblance. There seems in them usually a great tendency to dropsical swellings; and this consideration may serve to illustrate the nature of dropsy itself. — See also observations on Anæmia, by M. Halle, Journal de Medicine, tom. ix. and Edinburgh Medical and Surgical Journal, vol. iii.

dinary error of diet, and whether in fact there be in them any acrimony of the blood to be corrected, or altered texture to be resolved, is not very easy to determine.   If the general circumstances of the distemper have made such a state probable in the opinion of many able physicians, it is rendered more particularly so by the discovery of the coagulable nature of the urine, which would argue at least an altered texture of the lymph, and possibly some new saline matters favouring its solution.   These opinions, if fully proved, would lead to a beautiful simplicity of cure; a persuasion of their possible truth may induce us to look with a favourable eye, particularly in cachectic cases, on those mild, almost dietetic, remedies, which correct whilst they evacuate, or rather evacuate by correcting, and to which mineral and violent drugs have perhaps too universally succeeded.

SECTION V.

Of Tonic Remedies; Peruvian Bark, Chaly-beates, Bitters.

WHEN the evacuants, from whatever class they have been selected, have answered their purpose, it is usual to follow with considerable activity the last indication, viz. to prevent a relapse by tonics.

Of these the principal, and the only very powerful, are the cinchona and the preparations of iron. They have been given with various success, whilst the dropsy has still subsisted. In the early stages they are generally very injurious; in the more advanced, sometimes a great loss of tone is produced by severe sloughing ulcers of the lower extremities, or the flow of serum from scarified wounds. If a dexterous exhibition of the Peruvian bark is at this time made, the patient is deluged with his own discharges, and recovers.

After the water is evacuated, the urine either continues tinged with albumen or not. In the former case, the exhibition of tonics is a matter of great delicacy, since, if given too soon, they will most assuredly reproduce the disease in its most aggravated shape. In the latter, particularly after the use of fox-glove, they generally confirm the strength, and put the patient out of any fear of a relapse. This plan is, however, to be pursued more cautiously after an hydrothorax, than any other form of dropsy, an inflammation of the membranes or signs of stricture being very apt to return. The previous existence of an anasarca, ascites, or even an hydrocephalus, forms no objection to it.

Sometimes an unsound viscus prevents the possibility of improving the general strength, or even clearing up the urinary discharge; and this symptom continues unaltered, notwithstanding the exhibition of the most approved tonics and evacuants. It is needless to add, that nothing favourable can occur in such a state.

I have used the term tonics generally;

and perhaps practitioners are too much in the habit of considering bark and steel as equivalent, where tone is wanted. In the present disorder it is far otherwise, bark being infinitely to be preferred after the dropsy of young persons, of acute disease, and of sound stamina, steel being suited to a vitiated rather than a feeble habit, and indicated more by a pale sallow complexion and want of red colour in the blood, as shown by the paleness of the lips, than by any other signs. I must acknowledge myself to have had much more experience of the benefit of the former, than of the latter, after these dropsies.

Perhaps, where the tonics above-mentioned are thought too heating, mild bitters may be tried with advantage.

SECTION VI.

Of Mercury, and the Combination of it with Squills and Digitalis. — Conclusion.

I⊤ remains to say something of the use of mercury. Dr. Willan, in his work on Diseases of the Skin, has remarked, that if he could only point out the proper application of mercury in those complaints, the end of his publication would not be entirely lost. In dropsy this mineral is given in a manner equally indiscriminate and in larger doses, and with such opposite success, as to make it highly desirable that its exhibition should, if possible, be not conjectural, but defined and guided by some plain rules. Some firmness of the general habit will, I believe, be the best encouragement to it; and although there may be many other circumstances capable of denoting such a state, which have been justly pointed out by Dr. Maclean to be the same as call for the use of squills, yet I think the characters of the urine are the most easily understood, and the least liable to any misconception. If that discharge errs chiefly by want of dilution, the presence of bile, &c., mercury is likely to render great service in the obstructions which are probably present, particularly those of the liver, and also to prove a true diuretic ; and the swellings never pass off so readily and freely, as when the gums become affected. If, on the contrary, the habit is so depraved, that the coagulable part of the blood already passes off by the kidneys, the operation of this mineral is obviously very equivocal and hazardous. I do not so much from my own individual experience assert, that it can under no circumstances resolve such an obstruction, as I am confident, that there are many strong arguments against its use, and many cases in which it does great injury.

1st. Mercury is itself calculated to produce this discharge, since the dropsies that have followed its employment have been generally of this species, and a simple dropsy has been converted into it during a salivation.

2dly. Under the use of the submuriate of

mercury a bloody sediment has appeared, in addition to the presence of serum.

3dly. In some habits a remarkable buffiness of the blood follows mercurial courses, to which state there is already too great a tendency in the disease of which we are treating. Can we expect that these courses should both excite and remove such a tendency?

4thly. Mercury is singularly hostile to the constitution in any approach towards scurvy; and the dropsy with coagulable urine in many symptoms nearly resembles the land-scurvy, if indeed it be not under such circumstances entirely the same disorder.

5thly. It often rapidly affects the gums, and with great distress; and I have never seen a salivation of itself cure the disease, but often much aggravate it.

To these objections I have to oppose only the following very meagre facts; that in a moderately strong person labouring under this dropsy, a salivation was raised by friction; on the very evening on which the gums first became sore, some diuresis came on, and the urine, then discharged, was more devoid of serum than usual ; but this good effect was not permanent, although the salivation was continued ; I therefore was disposed to think the coincidence in some degree accidental. In some others mercury and digitalis combined produced a cure, whilst the gums were slightly affected. Calomel likewise is very commonly joined with digitalis after scarlatina and in the hydrothorax, and they apparently relieve. If this and a sort of indefinite experience of the benefits of mercury in dropsy should induce any one to try salivations in this form of it, he will of course select for his first experiments those habits which are most remote from an entire cachexy ; and it is obvious that his results will be very inconclusive, if he at the same time exhibits digitalis.

Doubts likewise may be entertained, how far true bilious symptoms may admit of the submuriate of mercury in this disease ; I am more fearful that the slightly sallow colour brought on by a deficiency of blood may be mistaken for the signs of an irregular bile.

There is one species of dropsical effusion,

z

against which the whole strength of such courses is generally directed, with what a melancholy result, the experience of the unfortunate parents can best say. I allude to the hydrocephalus internus. There are perhaps no cases more satisfactory or more creditable to the practitioner, than those fevers of children with an oppression of the head, in which a bold use of calomel brings off black discharges, and the patient from that moment recovers. Without inquiring here, whether the hydrocephalus is not thus cured which never existed, I wish to confine myself to that dropsy, when distinguished by the presence of serum in the urine ; and to state, that, after scarlatina, the tendency to this alarming conversion is increased under the use of mercurial purges ; that during the exhibition of two grains of the submuriate of mercury alone every night, which did not purge, the anasarca has disappeared and the head become affected ; and that there cannot be a more hopeless or more painful task, than that of submitting to the miserable routine of salivating such patients. On the other hand, digitalis assisted by active topical depletion has entirely succeeded. I look at the former of these two last remedies, as the most certainly of any, and the most rapidly, correcting the habit ; and to the latter, as necessary in the mean time to divert. the attack from the important organ on which it falls. And for this purpose the derivation should be made as speedily as possible, not only by taking blood from the temporal artery, where that operation is justifiable, but by an external inflammation suddenly raised. A bladder of hot water applied to the head, previous to laying on a large cap-blister, would contribute something towards the suddenness of this effect. Mustard-cataplasms quickened with oil of turpentine might likewise very advantageously be placed on the feet, as I suppose any thing so volatile could not be well applied to the head itself. The effects of these cataplasms when laid on the chest in the typhoid pneumonia, a disorder not uncommon in this county, are very striking. They produce within an hour excessive pain, and an inflammation entering much more into the true skin than that which is excited by cantharides ; and I have seen them beyond

any doubt rescue from impending suffocation.   I consider them well worthy the
attention of the practitioner in all internal
inflammations, where bleeding is limited.

Many physicians are fond of combining
squill calomel and digitalis, as a diuretic in
dropsy ; a practice often unsafe, and not
very decidedly possessing the merit even of
being consistent.   Digitalis greatly de-
presses the action of the heart and arteries,
and controuls the circulation ; and it seems
most unreasonable to believe, that its curative powers can be independent of such an
effect, or at least in any instance in contradiction to it.   On the other hand, mercury, if it does not pass off quickly, is
always exciting fever, and raising and hard-
ening the pulse.   In what errors of the
constitution are agents so very opposite
likely to be combined with advantage ?
Speaking from experience, where the urine
is coagulable and digitalis agrees, both the
others are, often at least, positively injurious; and the addition of them has this bad
effect besides, that by the sickness and
purging to which they are likely to contribute, they confuse the whole result, and

15

leave us in doubt what part of these bad symptoms is owing to the digitalis. If then we wish for the full effect of this remedy, it should be given as simply as possible, and not with those articles which may prematurely affect the stomach or bowels.

On the other hand, where the urine is foul and not coagulable and squills with calomel render service, I have on that very account made less trial of digitalis, and cannot speak of it from much experience. * Still further, should it be found by accurate experiment, that in some of those numerous cases, where they all, I fear, fail separately, they succeed when combined, it will certainly be a great improvement in the treatment of the disease. It is to the indiscriminate employment of this combination on all occasions that I principally object. Where relapse is so common, particularly in the hydrothorax, it is of great

---

* Two cases have lately occurred to me, which make me think it probable, that the efficacy of digitalis in dropsy is not confined to a coagulable state of the urine.

z 3

consequence to exhaust the strength of the patient as little as possible, and to ascertain precisely to what we have to trust. These objects are certainly more readily accomplished by simplicity of prescription, than by any doubtful additions. And it is above all things necessary that we should know better than we yet do, what these remedies can effect separately, and where they are safe, before we undertake so freely to combine them.

The crystals of tartar have been mentioned as particularly applicable to general dropsy, where the urine is coagulable as well as foul, and mild laxatives are wanted; I must however acknowledge, that I have no reason whatever to object to the use of this article as a mild aperient, where the urine is not coagulable, as in Chapter IV. Dr. Maclean speaks of it and the squills, as suited to the same constitutions.

I have now concluded my observations on the subject of dropsy, not, I trust, without leaving a conviction in the mind of the reader favourable to the general importance of the inquiry. Whatever difference of opinion may exist as to the nature or cure of that extraordinary symptom so often mentioned in the course of these remarks, it is impossible to overlook in it signs of a deviation from the healthy state. Neither can it be denied, that the disorder thus denoted materially differs from other forms of dropsy, however the general resemblance of the œdematous swellings may have been the means of confounding them. On these grounds I earnestly recommend it to the attention of every practitioner; and I am most confident, that his labour will soon be rewarded in the improved application of his remedies.

z 4

POSTSCRIPT.

THE third volume of Transactions of a Society for the Improvement of Medical and Chirurgical Knowledge, 1812, contains two valuable papers by Dr. Wells relating to dropsy ; one entitled, Observations on the Dropsy which succeeds Scarlet Fever ; the other, On the Presence of the red Matter and Serum of the Blood in the Urine of Dropsy which has not originated in Scarlet Fever. The above publication did not fall into my hands till long after this work was in the press, and too late to be noticed at all in the early part of it ; I have therefore purposely reserved what I had to say respecting it to this place, recommending to the reader at the same time a perusal of the papers themselves, as containing much and very accurate information on both the points on which they profess to treat, but particularly, I think, with regard to the symptoms of dropsy after scarlatina.

The suddenness of this disease, as described by Dr. Wells, the marks which he observed of peritoneal inflammation and pleurisy, the extreme danger so early as the third day, prove certainly much more than I have advanced in the preceding pages with regard to the acuteness and inflammatory nature of the attack.

In a large proportion of cases he found red blood to be deposited in the urine; in many more it was foul when made, and threw down a lymph or mucus; in all but two, and those slight cases, it was coagulable.

The urine was examined by Dr. Wells in one hundred and thirty persons affected with dropsy from other causes than scarlatina; of whom ninety-five were males, and thirty-five females. * In three of these red blood was observed; and in seventy-eight,

* The author informs us, that the male patients at St. Thomas's Hospital, where the observations were chiefly made, are so much more numerous than the females, as to prevent any conclusion from these numbers.

of whom sixty were males and eighteen females, serum was detected by the heat of
boiling water, or by nitrous acid. *   The
second of these tests he considers to be occasionally necessary,   as sometimes urine
does not, when it is made to boil, give any
precipitate, whilst that effect is readily produced by nitrous acid.   This want of
coagulation he attributes, apparently with
much reason, to a deficiency of salts in the
urine ; since if to serum in a state too
diluted for coagulation by heat, but still
capable of being coagulated by nitrous,

* I must caution the reader against considering the
number of cases related under each head in the preceding pages, as bearing any exact proportion to the number of dropsies with coagulable or uncoagulable urine
which have occurred to me.   I selected the most important.   Many examples of ascites with diseased liver
are omitted, where the urine was not coagulable ; and
many cases, where the urine had that property are
passed over, which were either not finished or illustrated nothing.   The second and third chapters are
however nearly exact in this respect.   Speaking from
memory, I believe that the urine has been serous, in
a very considerable majority of the important dropsies
that have occurred to me, and likewise that a majority
of those patients have been males ; as I think will be
found to be the case in dropsy generally.

acid, any neutral salts be added, heat likewise will occasion a precipitate. This observation shows the propriety of employing
nitrous acid whenever the test of heat fails ;
but the latter is infinitely superior for common purposes ; since it shows not merely
the existence of coagulable matter, but the
circumstances under which it does exist,
its quantity, and its tendency to separation, much more accurately than any other
test.

Amongst twenty-nine cases of anasarca
not symptomatic, were twenty-three with
urine containing serum ; in several, to a considerable extent. Of nine cases of anasarca, preceded by some debilitating disease,
as dysentery, ague, &c., in only two was
the urine at all coagulable. Of thirty-seven
cases of anasarca, preceded by cough and
dyspnœa, there was serum in the urine of
twenty-four. Of twenty cases of hydrothorax, serum in the urine of fourteen, in only
one to any considerable quantity. In four
encysted dropsies, three attended by anasarca, the urine contained no serum. Of
twenty-one cases of ascites, not preceded by
anasarca, there was a little serum in the

urine of seven.   In eight cases of ascites, preceded by diffused dropsy, it contained a very large proportion.

In twelve instances the urine was found to become solid, on being raised to the heat of boiling water ; in five it was firmly so, in seven a soft solid.

As serum more than twice diluted with water ceases to coagulate by heat, that mixture could not be used as a comparative test of the quantity of serum present in coagulable urine.   The author, therefore, substituted healthy urine for water, and finding that four parts of urine and one part of serum became solid by heat, he thought himself entitled to conclude with a tolerable degree of accuracy, that where dropsical urine barely forms into a solid mass, the serum constitutes about a fifth part of it ; once only the coagulum being unusually firm, he thought that serum made one-fourth of the mass.   The lesser quantities, as determined by a similar mode, appear to be very various, from 1-640th of the mass to 1-10th, 1-8th when the whole is converted into a semifluid jelly, 1-7th a firmer jelly and beginning to adhere to the phial, 1-6th a still firmer jelly, great part of which adheres to the phial. Agreeably to this estimate, he calculated that one patient passed four ounces of serum in the day, another five, another seven. For the further detail of these experiments I refer to the work itself.

The quantity of urine made daily amounted in one instance to ten pints, in some others to six pints. The appetite was sometimes great, the skin usually pale, the pulse large and frequent, with a tendency to diarrhœa, to hæmorrhages, and to a change of place in the external swellings.*

In order to ascertain how far the presence of serum in urine is peculiar to dropsy, Dr. Wells examined that secretion in many persons in health, and did not find serum in any, excepting in a very remarkable instance of a man, who, when dropsical, had discharged red blood as well as serum, and in whom, nine years after, whilst he was in apparent health and in a laborious employ-

* This change of the seat of dropsical swellings has been always mentioned as particularly attendant on scorbutic dropsies. See page 146.

ment, the urine became turbid on being boiled, and deposited a considerable quantity of curdy matter.

A similar examination was made in nineteen cases of acute disease. In fourteen of them the urine was altogether without serum, in four it had a very small quantity, in one about 1-160th.

Of eighty-five chronic cases, in fifty-four the urine had no serum, in twenty-five a very little, in one somewhat more, but likewise mixed with pus from a disease in the kidneys; in four who had been using mercury freely, rather a larger quantity.

On examining the urine in six patients before they began the use of mercury for the cure of syphilis, in five there was no serum, in the sixth a very small quantity. After a salivation continued for a fortnight, in the last mentioned the serum was much increased, in three others some was detected, and in two there was none. In one who became dropsical after a free use of mercury, the urine contained no serum; in three others a large quantity.

From these observations it is concluded, that urine containing a considerable quantity of serum, very rarely, if at all, occurs in any disease in this country except dropsy, and even in those very rare cases, has been induced by mercury.

In three instances, an examination was permitted after death. In the first the liver was enlarged and hardened, and there were some hydatids in the right kidney; in the second the right lung and diaphragm were inflamed, and the kidneys unusually thickened, and even changed in their structure; in the third, the liver was large and indurated, and the kidneys larger and softer than natural with several vesicles on their outside.

Dr. Baillie says of the tuberculated or scirrhous liver, that it is seldom larger. than in health; sometimes, he thinks, smaller; it is worthy of notice, that where the urine has been known to be coagulable, and the liver on examination has been found changed from its natural state, that change has tended generally to an increase of bulk, in one instance very remarkably so. *

* There is one exception to this in the dissections related in the preceding pages; in which the liver was

The kidneys likewise have been diseased in an unusual proportion in such dissections. In no less than three instances out of the eleven here referred to, viz. three in Dr. Wells's work and eight in mine, they were thickened or hardened, and even with a confused structure, in two or three containing hydatids or vesicles.

With respect to the cure, Dr. Wells derived no advantage from bark and steel; and squills digitalis and crystals of tartar did not seem to be so useful, as in other cases of dropsy. The tincture of cantharides was successful in two or three cases, and failed in two more.

In the same volume of the Transactions, is a paper containing an account of some changes from disease in the composition of human urine, by Mr. Brande. Two specimens of dropsical urine were examined by him at the request of Dr. Baillie. One of the parcels restored the colour of litmus paper reddened with vinegar, gave a considerable precipitate of albumen by the addi-

---

quite scirrhous but its bulk was not remarkable. See case, page 151.

tion of sulphuric acid, was found to contain hardly any urea, and deposited a sediment apparently lateritious, which, however, did not give any signs of uric acid on examination with nitric acid, but appeared to have been the rosaic acid of Proust.

The other parcel, from a man who had an ascites and diseased liver, ~ reddened litmus paper, afforded no signs of albumen, but gave a copious precipitate by tannin, and contained a much larger portion of urea, as ascertained by the usual method.

The absence of urea in the former of these parcels, which on common occasions constitutes a very large proportion, 19-20ths as Mr. Brande states, of the extractive matter, deserves much notice; as does also, its giving evidence of an excess of alkali, although we are not informed, how long after it was made, this experiment was tried.

A correct analysis of dropsical urine on an extensive scale, or even any thing approaching to correct, would undoubtedly form an important addition to the history of the disease; and it is much to be wished

A A

that the same gentlemen, who have so ably entered on this inquiry, would pursue it further.

———————

The remarks that I have made, in the preceding volume, on a purulent expectoration being sometimes attended by a coagulable state of the urine, have been incidental only, and perhaps briefly expressed.* I therefore add in this place, that it has appeared to me, both from dissections and symptoms in the living body, that a purulent expectoration so accompanied, is sometimes the result of that inflammatory habit, which, whilst it has attacked the serous membranes, and perhaps principally the pleuræ, has not wholly spared the body of the lungs ; in consequence of which, amidst the signs of a true dropsy, they suppurate and discharge. At other times, as far as I could collect from the statement of the patients, to an expectoration decidedly puru-

* See Page 214.

lent slight dropsical symptoms have been gradually added, with an urine somewhat coagulable; and in these there has been no true hectic nor colliquative discharges; but dropsy appears to have taken their place. An expectoration so circumstanced is not without hopes of cure; and I have lately had several cases of this kind under my management, in which, by abstaining from all evacuants, particularly calomel and digitalis, for the urine is not usually so scanty as to demand diuretics, by a moderately generous diet, some indulgence of the appetite, an allowance of fermented liquors, and the use of ten or fifteen grains of the pilulæ saponaceæ of the old dispensatories every night, the expectorated matter has gradually improved, and a recovery appears to be taking place.

There is indeed often in such patients a sallowness and bad colour, which give a suspicion of bilious complaints; and I have known it even suggested, particularly if the pain is of the right side or across the epigastrium, that the source of the expectorated matter is in the liver, which discharges itself through an ulcerated diaphragm.

A A 2

Allowing such a communication to be possible, it is, however, undoubtedly extremely rare, and seems to involve such a destruction of parts as precludes recovery; nor can it with the least appearance of truth be applied to explain the cases here described, which are certainly neither uncommon nor universally incurable. One point of treatment is agreed on by all reasonable practitioners, that if mercury is exhibited, it aggravates every symptom, and particularly alters for the worse the appearance of the expectorated matter. If, on the other hand, digitalis is given with a view of correcting the quality of the urinary discharge, it likewise fails in this effect, and the debility is aggravated. The principal chance of recovery seems to depend on supporting the general strength, not by bark and steel, but by a moderately liberal diet. I have also thought that the superacetate of lead, in the quantity of three or four grains daily, has had a favourable effect; and occasionally a light bitter.

Whilst finishing these papers, I was consulted by a poor man, who gave me the following account of his illness ; that about six weeks since, in very perfect health, he had been dancing at a fair in this neighbourhood, and walked home in the middle of the night, greatly overheated, and in a most severe rain. To that cause he attributed an attack, which in a few days became very evident, of general dropsy, attended by cough, and some pain of the chest. All those symptoms were greatly aggravated, when I saw him. The œdema was soft, the scrotum particularly distended, the bowels costive, and the abdomen bloated. His urine was scanty, grew speedily foul, and deposited a sediment resembling mucus in its appearance. It barely reddened the infusion of litmus within two hours after it was made, about twelve hours after had lost that property, and soon grew very fœtid. Exposed to heat at the same time with serum of the blood from a healthy person, it grew rather turbid before the serum thickened, viz. at about 150°, and at 160° was uniformly opaque and milky, and when forced a little further, but never so high as 190°, broke into soft white curds, mixed with a very little fluid. The serum became a pretty firm solid at 165°, and differed further from the coagulated urine, by being much less opaque.

A delay that occurred in finishing the Appendix, enabled me to subjoin to it, in the first edition, an account of the termination of the above case, which I now take the opportunity of transferring to this place.

I tried the infusion of digitalis with some hopes of success; but even in moderate doses it brought on a diarrhœa, which tincture of opium with difficulty checked. The tincture of squills every way disagreed.*

* In speaking of the liquid preparations of squills, and of the increase of their dose by drops, p. 76, I had particularly in my contemplation the tincture of squills; and as it is sometimes convenient and safe to entrust the increase of dose to the discretion of the patients, that form of prescription must, perhaps in some degree, be retained; there are, however, many great objections to it; and it should, as much as possible, be laid aside, particularly in drugs which affect life: since the nature of the fluid, the size of the phial, the thickness of its lip, even its cleanness, have an effect on the size

Crystals of tartar likewise affected the bowels violently; and the swellings increased. He became dull, unwilling to move, sleepy, confined himself almost to his bed, lay down nearly horizontally, had very little cough, with hardly any pain of the chest, and eat heartily. His extreme sensibility to cold was very striking; there was likewise great deficiency of red colour in the skin and lips, and such a feebleness of the circulation, that I really despaired of doing any good by blood-letting. In this state he continued nearly a month, when he was brought to the Hospital, and whilst remaining in the hall for admission felt some shiverings. In the evening a slight

of the drop, too considerable to be neglected. In reducing the drops of this tincture to minims, it will probably be sufficient for practical purposes to consider the minim as equal to two drops. On the other hand, the size of a drop of vinegar of squill is larger, and, approaches nearer to water; which circumstance, if overlooked, may occasion some confusion. With regard to the tincture of digitalis a similar caution, when converting drops into minims, is still more important, since, according to Mr. Shuttleworth's experiments, a drop of that preparation is even less than one of simple proof spirit.

erysipelatous blush appeared on his breast,
with an intense soreness to the touch.   It
spread to the integuments of the abdomen,
and in two days he died.

The body was opened the next morning.
The viscera of the abdomen were generally
sound ; the liver quite natural, all the pe-
ritonæal membranes without a cloud.   The
kidneys were thought large, and in their
cortical part of a colour somewhat browner
and duller than usual.

In the thorax, the lungs were connected
to the ribs generally by very recent and soft
adhesions.   On examining them further, it
appeared, that the pleura costalis was lined
with a thin layer of red and soft lymph,
which, on being separated with care, left
the real membrane nearly smooth.   The
pleura pulmonalis was covered with a similar adventitious membrane, which admitted
of the most entire separation from it.   This
process was less complete on the left side
of the thorax, where likewise was about a
pint of bloody fluid.*   The lungs were ra-

* A most complete example of this double membrane was observed at the Lunatic Asylum a few weeks

ther overloaded with blood, but contained neither tubercle, nor defined hardness ;

since. A gentleman, who had been insane for some months, but was not suspected of pulmonary complaints till after his admission into the house, died suddenly within a fortnight after that period, in consequence of a very large hæmoptoe. During his short residence there, he had complained of no pain, had a quick pulse, an incoherent agitation of spirits, remarkable timidity mixed with violence, and almost every day some intervals of reason. An uncommon sense of coldness was very marked in him, so that he would lay himself down near the fire ; and he was observed to have a nightly cough with dark sputa.

On opening the body, besides the lungs being found full of small vomicæ, the left lung was invested with a very thick adventitious membrane, separable in long strips somewhat resembling buff. Another membrane in close adhesion with this lined the pleura costalis, not so easily separable and redder ; and at the lower part, where the lung usually moves on the diaphragm, the natural surfaces were separated from each other by a double covering of this sort, closely adhering, and each more than 2-10ths of an inch in thickness. The pleura of the diaphragm was hardened and inflamed, and lymph was deposited between it and that muscle.

The abdomen was entirely sound ; the brain likewise, a perfect example of healthy structure and natural state of the vessels. This was, probably, therefore, a case of paraphrenitis, though less acute than those described by Boerhaave and others. It was under the more immediate care of my friend Dr. Daniell, by whose obliging permission I insert it here. To him, trachea inflamed ; heart small, natural ; in the pericardium, about three ounces of clear fluid.

The membranes of the brain were entirely free from inflammation ; and its lateral ventricles contained hardly any fluid ; but its substance was remarkably soft, although the body was opened not above nineteen hours after death and was free from putrefaction.

Besides the watery serum which flowed from the incisions made in the cellular membrane of the body, it was in many places loaded with an effusion half-coagulated, soft, and of a gelatinous appearance. Underneath the seat of the erysipelas on the breast, this was interspersed with many minute coagula of blood.

On the above dissection little comment is necessary. We find an urine, which becomes nearly solid by heat, to be attendant

the public are much indebted for his exertions in the medical department of the institution, at a time particularly when such charities were less generally known than they begin to be at present; and the excellent arrangements, which he has greatly contributed to make, give certainly to his present colleague duties of a comparatively easy nature.

on effusions evidently inflammatory, without any very marked disease of the viscera themselves. It is obvious from the difficulty with which the stomach bore remedies, that if any treatment could have saved life, it would have been venæ-section in the early stage.

APPENDIX.

ON THE ANGINA PECTORIS.

THE following cases appear to be correct examples of the Angina Pectoris ; and I hope, that the dissections annexed to them will not be unacceptable to the reader.

The interest that has been excited by that remarkable disease is reasonably due to its very singular symptoms, and the great ability with which Dr. Heberden first described them. Some obscure mention of them is indeed found in preceding authors ; but it is such only as is sufficient to shew, that this illustrious physician copied from nature rather than from his predecessors, and drew the picture more faithfully.

There is one circumstance alone, in which the novelty of the subject necessarily rendered his information partial and

2

inconclusive. I allude to the appearances ascertained by dissection. This deficiency has been in a great measure supplied by succeeding writers; and the injury sustained by the great organs of circulation has been usually found much more severe and extensive, than Dr. Heberden seems to have suspected.

With regard to the cure, almost every thing remains to be done; but we need not despair of at length obtaining it, when we shall have determined more precisely the nature of these changes, and the constitutional disorders in which they originate.

For the first case, with the remarks annexed to it, I am indebted to my late friend and colleague Dr. Parr, whose high professional character gives them a considerable authority, and which I have thought it right to communicate in his own words.

CASE I.

" J. S. ætat. 64, a stout man, with a full " and short neck, not inactive, nor subject

" to any particular complaint in the former
" part of his life.   About eight years before
" his death he was confined for some time
" in prison for debt, and soon after his re-
" lease was seized with a pain at the lower
" part of the sternum, extending over his
" breast, and down his arms to the tops of
" his fingers, together with great oppression
" of breathing.   In a few minutes all the in-
" convenience was removed, which was so
" slight, that it was little noticed, and attri-
" buted to rheumatism.   In the course of
" six years, the attacks gradually increas-
" ing, had become very violent, and came
" on chiefly, while walking, but ceased on
" stopping for a few minutes.   Some months
" afterwards they awakened him in the mid-
" dle of the night, and at length occurred
" on almost every exertion.   In addition
" to the former symptoms, the fingers dur-
" ing the attack were benumbed, the sto-
" mach swelled, and he felt a violent pain
" at the heart.   The recurrence of the pa-
" roxysms was irregular, their return not
" apparently influenced by the weather;
" and riding as well as walking occasion-

" ally produced them, as did likewise par-
" ticularly the straining to procure an eva-
" cuation.

" As the disease appeared to be what Dr.
" Heberden called angina pectoris, twenty-
" five drops of laudanum were given at
" night; and on the attack of a paroxysm,
" some nervous drops, with laudanum, tinc-
" ture of castor, and volatile aromatic spirit.
" To obviate costiveness and to discharge
" water, which appeared to be accumulat-
" ing in the chest, the cream of tartar was
" given in moderately large doses. Under
" this plan the fits were less frequent and
" violent, and their duration shorter. The
" cremor tartari soon lost its effect; and
" pills with equal parts of soap and aloes
" were substituted for them. A blister also
" was applied to the part of the sternum
" where the fits commenced. This remedy
" appeared to remove their apparent source
" from the sternum to the middle of the
" biceps muscle; but this continued for a
" short time only; and their origin was
" soon removed to the upper part of the
" sternum, just under the clavicles. Cop-
" per being at that time a favourite remedy

" in nervous paroxysms, a quarter of a grain
" of cuprum ammoniacum was given three
" times a day.   For the first three days
" after taking this medicine, he had no fit ;
" a circumstance which had not occurred
" for three years.   The paroxysms however
" returned, and continued to the period of
" his death, which was at last very sudden.

" On dissection, the thyroid gland was
" found greatly enlarged, seemingly from
" air in the cellular texture.   Near the ster-
" num the lungs adhered to the pleura, and
" they did not collapse when exposed to the
" air.   Their substance was sound ; but in
" the bronchia nearly three quarts of a
" dark-coloured bloody fluid were disco-
" vered; and in the cavities of the chest
" were two quarts of serum.   The arch of
" the aorta was enlarged to at least double
" its usual size, and thickly set with small
" ossifications.   The valves were nearly
" closed, and the interstices between their
" edges and the artery were filled with small
" irregularly shaped bones.   Little pieces
" of bone were interspersed in the muscular
" substance of the heart, and the carneæ
" columnæ were remarkably hard.   The ar-

" teries, which arise from the aorta, were
" somewhat enlarged.

" I shall subjoin some remarks at that
" time suggested to Dr. Heberden on the
" subject. Is it not probable, that the ap-
" pearances here, and in other cases on dis-
" section, shew only the effects of the dis-
" ease, and that the attack was at first no
" organic or inflammatory affection of the
" vessels near the heart, but partook of the
" nature of a spasm? Almost all the symp-
" toms are explicable on the supposition
" of a contraction of the arch of the aorta,
" or the arteries that go to the arm; and
" we know that spasm exists at times in all
" the muscles which carry on the vital
" and involuntary functions. This view
" will likewise point out the source of the
" changes discovered on dissection. The
" effusion in the trachea was probably the
" fatal stroke. These, however, are mere
" conjectures.

" This case occurred about the year
" 1774."

CASE II.

William Duffell, a sailor of a robust make and very open chest, aged 65, was admitted into the Devon and Exeter Hospital under my care in September, 1798.

He was subject to very severe attacks of pain in the region of the heart, attended by the most dreadful anxiety and sense of faintness. They were brought on by the slightest exercise, and obliged him to remain perfectly still for some minutes, when the pain moved towards the left shoulder and clavicle, but never down either arm, and he became easy. Eructations always accompanied and in some degree relieved them.

At other times he was free from any uneasiness, lay in bed on either side without the least degree of orthopnœa, and could take a pretty full inspiration. His pulse was usually about 80 in the minute, rather quick and thrilling.

He had formerly suffered much from rheumatism; his present complaints attacked him about eight months before his admission, and seemed to come on rather suddenly and severely, being attended at first by a symptom which in the progress of the disease almost disappeared, fits of suffocation, as he called it, after his first sleep ; in which he was obliged to go to the open window for relief.

I directed for him no remedies of any importance, except an issue on the inside of his thigh ; and he had been in the Hospital but a few days, when the mere effort of putting on his coat without assistance produced a very violent paroxysm, which lasted nearly an hour, and during which I saw him. His countenance was much shrunk and contracted; his respiration, though certainly not more rapid than ordinary, yet carried on with great anxiety and distress ; the pulse very feeble and intermittent ; the faculties of his mind unimpaired. The eructations were violent and incessant, and he encouraged them as giving some relief. He recovered from this fit, but two or three hours afterwards, whilst using some very slight exertion, fell down and expired instantly.

The body was opened the next day. We

found the abdominal viscera sound and in a natural state, except that there was more air than usual in the intestines ; most of the cartilages of the ribs ossified ; the external surface of the pericardium and all the anterior mediastinum somewhat overloaded with fat ; a small quantity of turbid water in the cavity of the pericardium ; the surface of the aorta, about the distance of an inch from the heart, slightly inflamed ; some small ossifications in the valves of both ventricles, and the muscular substance of the heart itself remarkably soft and flaccid ; the semilunar valves of the aorta sound, excepting two small ossified spots ; but the aorta itself, from the heart to the diaphragm, thickened and dilated, its inner surface lying in folds and wrinkles, with many ossifications between it and the muscular coat. At a little distance from the semilunar valves, there was a more considerable deposition of bone than in any other spot ; and an incipient ulceration of the inner membrane answering to the appearance of inflammation, mentioned above, in the external surface of the aorta. There was not a greater quantity of fluid than natural in the cavities of the thorax; the lungs were sound, but somewhat overloaded with blood, and connected to the pleura costalis by very extensive adhesions.

This case happened before the publication of Dr. Parry's very ingenious work on syncope anginosa, and the coronary arteries of the heart were not particularly examined.

CASE III.

This occurred to me at Totness, in the spring of 1807, and is as follows :

Peter Bastoe, ætat. 60, of a spare habit of body, narrow-chested, rather free in his mode of living and subject to rheumatism, had for more than twelve months before his death been liable to attacks of pain at the pit of the stomach, which after a few minutes passed off between the shoulders and down both arms as far as the elbows. A considerable uneasiness likewise ran downwards to the bladder, with a most distressing and irresistible inclination to make water. These paroxysms were originally produced by walking up hill, and afterwards by every little exertion of body and mind, and excess of diet. As the disease advanced, they became more frequent, and were excited by slighter causes, till at length they occasionally came on in bed, after his first sleep. At these times he was obliged to rise, and the strangury became particularly troublesome. Once, a very hearty meat-supper was the cause of the attack. It lasted two hours. He lay totally insensible, his respiration slow and nearly suspended, his pulse beating with the most extreme weakness and intermissions, and the urine flowing involuntarily. The next day, besides a good deal of languor and debility, he had some cough; this symptom, however, was not usual to him. The severe nightly paroxysms were generally foretold by palpitations, and a smart stroke of the artery; but, during them, I understood him to be free from any sensation of that kind.

At other times his pulse was 80 in the

1

minute; and I observed nothing very remarkable in the stroke of the artery. He lay down easily in bed, and indifferently on either side, till within two months before his death, when he preferred the right side; and so free was he from any dyspnœa, that to the last, he was in the habit of playing the bassoon in public concerts. The pain in the arms was at first very marked, but rather decreased in its severity and extent, as the disorder advanced. I could not learn that he had had any obstructions of the urethra in the former part of his life; nor after repeatedly questioning him, did it so much appear to me, that these painful efforts to make water brought on the fit, as that they followed almost instantaneously the anxiety at the heart.

I considered it possible, however, that his symptoms might be connected with a calculus of the kidneys; and the medicines which I at first directed were given under that idea. But he derived no service from them. I was equally unsuccessful in my attempts to palliate the symptoms by opiates or any other means; and not many weeks after, whilst walking in the street, he complained of extreme faintness, dropt, and was taken up dead.

We were next day permitted to open the body. We found the substance of the lungs sound, but the left lung every where adhering pretty firmly to the pleura; no more than a natural quantity of fluid either in the right side of the thorax or pericardium; the heart large and fat, but very flaccid; the aorta, as it emerged from it, rather inflamed externally; the internal membrane, as far as the aorta descendens, in many places thickened and of an irregular surface, and with several spots of incipient ossification; the semilunar valves ossified, the bony deposition in one of them being nearly of the size of a common garden pea. and apparently sufficient to give considerable impediment to its action; the coronary arteries ossified. In the right coronary, for more than an inch from its origin, the deposition of bony matter, not from all sides uniformly towards the centre, but across the cavity from one side towards

the other, had been so great as very nearly
to obliterate its canal : the left was enlarged, and, as far as could be traced, its coats
were almost completely converted into
bone.   The other valves of the heart and
of the pulmonary artery were quite sound.

The viscera of the abdomen were natural ;
particularly in the kidneys, ureters, and
bladder, there was not the least appearance
of disease ; but I am unable to speak with
precision of that part of the canal beyond
the bladder.

CASE IV.

W. Sprague, ætat. 50, Hospital, 1810,
suffered from severe attacks of pain in the
region of the heart.   The commonest exertions produced it, but particularly walking
up hill, stooping, or costive discharges.   It
was attended by palpitations.   On resting,
it passed off in a few minutes upwards to
the shoulders, and down each arm as far as
the elbows, particularly the left.   At the

same time a kind of forcing pain ran rapidly downwards to the bladder, and ended in an irresistible inclination to make water. Such were his sensations of this kind, that it was very difficult to persuade him that he was not affected with the gravel, although certainly none ever appeared in his urine; and he often told me that he was free from strangury, except during the paroxysm. He occasionally found some relief by leaning forward and raising his arms above his head against the bed-post, as if to give his chest greater expansion. I had no opportunity of seeing him in those attacks, and therefore cannot speak to the state of the circulation during them; but he repeatedly said, that they were attended by palpitations of the heart, and by a difficulty of breathing; the exact nature of that distress he was wholly unable to describe. He laboured habitually under some degree of pyrosis; the pulse was generally 80, quick and thrilling; and there was a very constant expression of anxiety in the countenance.

He had been much troubled with a chronic and painful rheumatism till within the last twelve months ; since which his chest had been attacked ; and it is remarkable, as in Duffell's case, that at first he used to suffer most severely in the night, being waked from a sound sleep by a sort of painful spasm ; after a few weeks, his rest in general ceased to be disturbed in this way.

I directed him the pills of soda and soap, as apparently most suited to the circumstances of the attack. An issue was also opened in one of his thighs. But the hard labour, which he persisted in going through, perpetually renewed his complaint ; and his symptoms increased rather rapidly. One night after eating something difficult of digestion, he was waked by a severe paroxysm, which continued for some hours, when he expired.

On opening the body, we found a great deal of fat in the anterior mediastinum ; the lungs quite sound ; about a pint of pale serum on the left side of the thorax, somewhat less on the right ; no adhesions ; in the pericardium no more fluid than natural ; one white lymphy spot on the surface of the heart ; the surface of the great vessels rather inflamed, the right ventricle and pulmonary artery sound ; valvulæ mitrales somewhat ossified ; aorta thickened and most completely covered as far as the arch with very solid ossifications, round and upon which in some places the inner membrane had ulcerated. The ossification was particularly hard and thick in a spot very near one of the semilunar valves ; but the valves themselves were quite free from any degeneration of this kind.

The coronaries were dissected for many inches, and their canals laid open ; they were found in a natural state, except two very small and thin white spots or rudiments of ossifications in the left coronary, about an inch from its origin, which did not produce the least unevenness or rigidity in the inner surface ; and if any such changes can be said to be harmless, these were undoubtedly so. Their size was very minute, not one-tenth of an inch in diameter.

In the abdomen the intestines were much filled with air ; but every part was sound in its structure; I speak particularly of the urinary organs, which were very carefully examined.

CASE V.

The following as an instance not common, of the disease being connected with external violence, will perhaps be deemed worthy the attention of the reader.

R. B. ætat. 60, a coachman, three months before he consulted me, received a violent blow from the pole of a carriage, which forcing him against a wall produced some little contusion of the surface of the chest, and an internal pain, for which he was blooded, and used a liniment. He continued affected in his breathing on motion, and two months afterwards, whilst he was pitching some hay into a loft, he felt a violent pain in the region of the heart spreading rapidly to the left arm, with faintness and inability of movement. A similar paroxysm came on several successive nights, waking him with an approach to deliquium and great anxiety.   It continued to return on every exertion, and went off only by rest.   But after he had quitted his situation, and was liable to less fatigue, the attacks became milder.

Twenty years since he suffered severely from rheumatism, and after his first accident, what the apothecary considered to be gout appeared for two or three days in both his feet.

He received some advantage from very mild laxatives, and the keeping a seton open on his chest ; and by avoiding the occasional causes, and using great abstinence, has now for several years regained a firm state of health.

Previously to considering the anatomical evidence furnished by these cases, I wish to make some observations, suggested by the symptoms.

1st. The symptom of palpitation mentioned in the fourth case, is not perhaps generally present in the angina pectoris ; but it seems to make no material alteration in the character of the disease. Palpitations are often rather a diminished than an increased action of the heart, the ineffectual and feeble efforts of a distressed organ. They not only precede and are observed in the intervals of syncope both from a nervous and organic cause, but are sometimes united with a total cessation of the pulse at the wrist. Of the former fact, I was lately witness to an example, in a patient affected with angina pectoris, who felt palpitations and tremblings of the heart, from slight causes, but never in the paroxysm itself. Of the latter a remarkable instance is given in Deidier des Tumeurs, which Dr. Parry quotes from Senac as a case of ossified coronaries. The symptoms are as follows :

A lady, ætat, 84, had been troubled for some time with a singular oppression at the chest, not connected with dyspnœa. She had a constant distressing palpitation below the ensiform cartilage, and returns from time to time of paroxysms characterised by the apprehension of instant death, by the total cessation of the pulse at the wrist, cold extremities, a perfect freedom of the head, and a great increase of the palpitations.

The semilunar valves were found ossified; the aorta contracted at its curvature, and ossified from its origin to its termination in the iliacs; the same process had extended to its branches, especially the left coronary, which was hard, cartilaginous, and half ossified. The other circumstances, both of the case and dissection, I pass over, as not throwing any particular light on the present subject. *

2d. The uncommon effect of the blister, in the case communicated to me by Dr. Parr, is well worthy of notice, and renders it highly probable, if such a proof were wanting, that a muscular spasm forms part of the complaint. It has been already mentioned in Dr. Duncan's Medical Commentaries, vol. iii.

3d. The pain of the arm appears to be very variable both in its extent and the time

---

* Deidier des Tumeurs, page 329. — See also Mr. Weldon's case, Medical and Physical Journal, vol. xvi. where palpitation is noticed as present in the paroxysm.

of its coming on. In some instances it is found to precede, in others to follow the fit ; it sometimes attacks both arms, as we see in case third and fourth, sometimes only the left, and it terminates in almost any spot from the insertion of the deltoid to the finger's ends. In the second case, it reached no farther than the clavicle and shoulder. When extending, however, as it usually does, it becomes a very important sign, which strongly arrests the attention of the patient by its singularity, often gives the first notice of the nature of the complaint, and may much assist the medical practitioner in forming his diagnostic.

4th. The strangury as it appeared in the third and fourth cases, is unusual, and has, I believe, been wholly overlooked by medical writers. But Lord Clarendon, in the *History of his own Life,* records a similar fact respecting his father, and in terms so just and descriptive, that I have subjoined the account in his own words. * The

* " His father had long suffered under an indisposi-
" tion (even before the time his son could remember)
" which gave him rather frequent pains, than sickness ;
" and gave him cause to be terrified with the expect-

c c

circumstances in which it differs from the cases above mentioned, the reader will be at no loss to discover, and will probably attribute that difference to the existence of some disorder in the urinary organs themselves.

Dr. Parry has stated this disease to par-

" ation of the stone, without being exercised with the
" present sense of it : but from the time he was sixty
" years of age, it increased very much, and four or five
" years before his death, with circumstances scarce
" heard of before, and the causes whereof are not yet
" understood by any physician; he was very often, both
" in the day and the night, forced to make water, sel-
" dom in any quantity, because he could not retain it
" long enough, and in the close of that work, without
" any sharp pain in those parts, he was still and con-
" stantly seized on by so sharp a pain in the left arm,
" for half a quarter of an hour, or near so much, that
" the torment made him as pale (whereas he was other-
" wise of a very sanguine complexion) as if he were
" dead ; and he used to say, ' that he had passed the
" ' pangs of death, and he should die in one of those
" ' fits;' as soon as it was over, which was quickly, he
" was the cheerfullest man living ; eat well such things
" as he could fancy, walked, slept, digested, conversed
" with such a promptness and vivacity upon all argu-
" ments (for he was *omnifariam doctus*) as hath been
" seldom known in a man of his age : But he had the
" image of death so constantly before him in those con-

take always of the nature of a syncope. And undoubtedly when the paroxysm has amounted to any degree of severity and immediate danger, these signs have usually been very obvious. Not only the pulse has indicated it, but the partial cessation of breathing *, the shrunk countenance, the cold extremities, and that remarkable sen-

---

" tinual torments, that for many years before his death, " he always parted with his son, as to see him no more; " and at parting still showed him his will, discoursing " very particularly, and very cheerfully of all things " he would have performed after his death. When he " had nearly completed his seventieth year, he, one " day, whilst at church, found himself a little pressed " as he used to be, and therefore thought fit to make " what haste he could to his house, and was no sooner " come thither into a lower room, than having made " water, and the pain in his arm seizing upon him, he " fell down dead, without the least motion of any limb. " The suddenness of it made it apprehended to be an " apoplexy, but there being nothing like convulsions, " or the least distortion or alteration in the visage, it is " not like to be from that cause; nor could the physi- " cians make any reasonable guess from whence that " mortal blow proceeded." Vol. i. page 16.

* In one patient whom I several times saw in the paroxysm, the pulse was 40, weak and interrupted, and he felt conscious, that the act of breathing required a voluntary effort.

sation of dying, which Seneca well expresses, when he says, *aliud, quicquid est,
ægrotare, est ; hoc est, animam agere.* The
faculties of the mind, on the other hand,
often remain unimpaired ; and this combination of symptoms, so unusual in syncope,
forms altogether the most distressing spec-
tacle that can be well imagined. There is
likewise great pain in the region of the
heart, attended sometimes by a remarkable soreness in the affected spot. The
pain always, in some degree, stretches
towards the left arm, often to both, even
downwards through the abdomen to the
bladder, and, as I once observed, down
the loins to the outside of both thighs and
legs ; but the extent of this sympathy
varies much, and must be expected to do
so, according to the predisposition of the
patient, and the exact nature of the organic
injury. Now and then an entire insensibility, with total loss of pulse, has taken
place. In many of those shorter and less
intense attacks, which medical persons do
not commonly witness, it is probable that
the same character prevails, though in a
less degree. I must add, however, that if

I can at all trust the statement of a patient
in his own case on such a subject, very
strong palpitations, and a smart stroke of
the artery, have preceded and even foretold severe nightly deliquia * ; and where
this fit may be strictly said to begin, may
admit of doubt ; are not these different
states rather parts of one great paroxysm,
commencing with an increase, and termi-
nating with a failure of the circulation ?
The syncopes, from an organic cause, have
been remarked often to possess this character,
long before the angina pectoris received
its name ; and it is worthy of notice, that
even in the true and acknowledged form
of that disease, the muscle of the heart
has not always been found in the same
condition, but in one instance emaciated,
soft, and rotten †, and in another large,
very hard, and strong ‡ ; in a third, the
left ventricle was remarkably strong and
thick. § These opposite changes hardly

---

* See Case III.
† Memoirs of London Medical Society, vol. i. Dr.
Johnstone's case.
‡ Morgagni Epistol. xxvi. Article 31.
§ Medical Transactions, vol. iii. — Dr. Heberden's.

seem compatible with an entire similarity
of diseased action during life.   In the first
instance, there is reason to suppose that
this organ was habitually very deficient
in force, and badly nourished ;   in the
two last, it must have been at least well
nourished, and often probably too active,
or exerting an activity suited to some unusual resistance.

Having endeavoured to ascertain what
constitutes the fit of angina pectoris, the
next question is, what causes it ; and upon
this head, the information derived from
dissection is strikingly uniform.   I am very
far indeed from denying that exceptions
have occurred, and may occur again; but
looking at the mass of evidence, and not
at the exceptions, the prevalence of an
ossification somewhere about the origin of
the aorta can hardly escape us.   I will as
briefly as possible enumerate the principal
appearances in these dissections, and shall
follow Dr. Parry's opinion with regard to
the genuineness of the disease, as far as his
publication extends, i. e. to the thirteenth
case.

1st Case. Morgagni Epistle xxvi. art. 31.—Aorta dilated and ossified, heart large, and very hard and strong.

2d. Medical Transactions, vol. iii. Dr. Heberden; dissection by Mr. J. Hunter. — A few specks of beginning ossification of the aorta, left ventricle of the heart remarkably firm and quite empty. Adhesion of the lungs to the pleura on the left side.

3d. Medical Transactions, vol. iii. Dr. Wall. — Heart very large and fat; a pint of water in the pericardium; semilunar valves of the aorta perfectly ossified and immoveable; aorta considerably enlarged, and in some degree ossified.

4th and 5th. Medical Observations and Inquiries, vol. v. Dr. Fothergill. · In one of these instances, besides water in the chest and accumulation of fat in the mediastinum, there was near the apex of the heart a white spot of the size of a sixpence, like a cicatrix. In the other, the muscular substance of the heart unusually pale, and in many places, having the appearance of incipient ossification; the valvulæ mitrales and aorta slightly ossified;

and the coronaries completely converted into bone.

6th. Duncan's Medical Commentaries, vol. iii. Dr. Percival. — Liver, particularly the left lobe, full of hard white tumours; stomach scirrhous, where it came in contact with the liver; heart and its vessels sound.

7th. Memoirs of the London Medical Society, vol. i. Dr. Johnstone. — The heart remarkably soft and flaccid, and easily admitting the finger to pass through its substance.

8th. Memoirs of the London Medical Society, vol. iv. Dr. Black. — Coronaries completely ossified; left auricle remarkably thin; aorta much dilated, so as to appear rather like a bag than an artery, and resembling in its substance white leather.

9th. Home's Life of Mr. John Hunter. — On examining the body of that very eminent anatomist, who died with decided symptoms of the disease; there were adhesions of the lungs to the pleura on the left side; pericardium thickened; heart unusually small; spots of lymph on its surface; its muscular substance very pale and loose; coronary arteries converted into bony tubes; valvulæ mitrales ossified in many places; incipient ossification in the semilunar valves of the aorta, aorta enlarged, and its inner membrane covered with white spots.

10th, 11th, 12th, 13th. Dr. Parry on Syncope Anginosa.

In the first (by Dr. Jenner), the symptoms of which are not detailed, but said generally to be those of angina pectoris; coronaries ossified.

Second (by Mr. Paytherus). Accumulation of fat in the mediastinum; pericardium inflamed; coats of the coronaries thickened, approaching to a cartilaginous state; their inner surface incrusted with lymph, which was traced and drawn out from their smallest ramifications; heart remarkably empty; in the bottom of the right ventricle an oval sloughy spot; coats of the aorta thickened in two places, and several white spots in its inner membrane.

Third, Semilunar valves slightly ossified;

aorta considerably enlarged; coronaries ossified.

Fourth, One of the semilunar valves of the aorta ossified; aorta dilated, and somewhat ossified; coronaries ossified.

14th. Memoirs of the London Medical Society, vol. vi. Dr. Black. — Coronaries completely ossified through their whole extent; aorta somewhat dilated.

15th. London Medical and Physical Journal, vol. xvi. Mr. Weldon. — Aorta thickened in its inner membrane in numerous spots, though without any bony deposit; coronaries sound; right lung filled with abscesses; left lung firmly adhering to the pleura and pericardium. This patient died from the effects of pneumonia, and had remained for some years before his death nearly free from the paroxysms of angina pectoris.

16th. London Medical and Physical Journal, vol. xvii. Mr. Ring. — Coronaries ossified; the mitral valves and semilunar valves of the aorta in different parts diseased and thickened, as if in an incipient state of ossification.

17th, 18th, 19th, 20th, related in this Appendix.

In the first, (Dr. Parr's) the heart and the aorta and its valves ossified, with considerable adhesions of the lungs ;

Second, Aorta enlarged and ossified, with universal adhesions of the lungs ;

Third, Aorta and its valves and coronaries ossified, with adhesions of the left lung ;

Fourth, Aorta ossified to a very great extent.

We may observe, that in three only of these twenty cases, Dr. Fothergill's first, Dr. Percival's, and Dr. Johnstone's, there was no appearance of ossification of the great vessels ; but in the first an hydrothorax, with fat in the mediastinum ; in the second an unsound liver ; in the third an unusual softness of the parietes of the heart.

The last of these states seems equally capable of producing an irregular and feeble action of that muscle, as any ossification can be ; and it was likewise very probably dependent on some obstruction of the coronaries not sufficiently noticed.

Of Dr. Percival's I shall only remark,

that it was briefly related, and but once seen by that physician ; and that there is an unsoundness of the liver or biliary congestion, which produces symptoms bearing a character of great resemblance to the angina pectoris, but, as far as I have seen, marked by a more active circulation, relievable in a great measure by venæ-section and vomits, as Dr. Percival's case was, and greatly injured by opiates. The practice, therefore, is very different, and the distinction between the two diseases should be precise.

In Dr. Fothergill's case, the changes found on dissection were certainly not sufficient to account for the symptoms ; and unless, as Dr. Parry has suggested, some ossification of the coronaries was overlooked, it must remain one of the exceptions before alluded to.

In all the remaining cases, there was some alteration of structure tending to ossification about the origin of the arterial system, in the greater part, very extensive. An unsoundness of the aorta in various degrees is the most frequent appearance, being found in fifteen of these seventeen cases. In nine the coronaries likewise were ascertained to be diseased ; in one the coronaries alone *; in several the valves and heart itself.

That when this process begins in the trunk of the aorta, it should spread to the branches, and particularly perhaps to the coronaries, was to have been expected. But dissection shows, that it has not always done so before the paroxysms have proved fatal. In two dissections, where the coronaries are not mentioned, and may have been overlooked, yet the heart was noticed as remarkably firm and well nourished. Morgagni's words, are *cor magnum potius et durum valde ac robustum* ; and in Dr. Heberden's case the left ventricle was said to be remarkably strong and thick ; a state very unlikely to coincide with a deficient nourishment, and habitual want of activity. Mr. Weldon asserts the coronaries to have been sound, in the instance which he relates ; and of the fourth case recorded in

* This case, where the coronaries alone were ossified, is the only one the symptoms of which are not accurately detailed, but said generally to be those of angina pectoris. See Parry on Syncope Anginosa, page 3.

this volume I shall only add, that those vessels were examined with the utmost care in the presence of very able judges, and no unsoundness of them was perceived, but the two small thickened spots before mentioned.

In two of these seventeen cases, Dr. Heberden's and Mr. Weldon's, the appearances are said to be slight, and not sufficient to satisfy the anatomists who conducted the dissection. What quantity of disorder is necessary in order to impair the action of any part, is not easily determined. It is still more difficult to make a correct allowance for the pain and disturbance, which often usher in changes of structure, and which may be very severe, even before the effect is produced satisfactory to the eye of an anatomist. Such small alterations of themselves, it will be allowed, do not prove a great deal; but when they are found in a suspected part, and are the least of a series of proofs, they acquire an additional value by that connection. We should likewise, in estimating such appearances, have some reference to the constitution of the patient, and allow it to be possible, as

it undoubtedly is, that circumstances, connected with that cause, may have given
activity to disorganizations apparently of
little consequence. Morbid anatomy presents us with the alterations of structure
only, and even those but imperfectly ;
during life there has been added something
peculiar to the living solid, which infinitely
modifies the effects of disordered structure.

Ossifications occur in those parts of the
arterial system principally, which are most
exposed to external impressions, or to the
increased impulses of the circulation. They
appear, however, not to be the effect of
these accidents simply ; since the causes
alluded to are very common, and indeed
almost universally occurring, whilst ossifications are at least comparatively rare. It is
reasonable therefore to suppose, that where
this change takes place to any considerable
extent, there has been a predisposition to
disease in the arteries themselves, perhaps
some feebleness of their original structure,
which makes them susceptible of injury
from slight violence. Sometimes this aneurismal diathesis extends to every artery in
the body ; and then no doubt can be enter-

tained of its connection with an internal cause. Even when the mischief is originally more local, its disposition to spread extensively to the neighbouring vessels is very remarkable; and the mode in which the unhealthy passes gradually into the healthy structure, argues something very different from a mere accidental injury.*

Some writers have connected these changes in the arterial system with a constitutional disorder.

Lancisi considers hypochondriacal, scorbutic, and syphilitic persons to be most liable to them.

---

* The late Dr. Parr, whose opinion on pathological questions is of high value, has suggested, as appears by some queries subjoined to the first case, that the original attack partakes in all instances of the nature of a spasm, and that the arteries, gradually only, become inflamed and ossified. In confirmation of the possibility of such a spasm, and of such gradual injury of the arterial coats by means of it, the late Mr. John Hunter's case occurs to me. During the first paroxysm which he ever suffered, and that a very severe one, brought on by anxiety of mind, the pain was seated about the pylorus; to which it may be added that calculi were found in the gall-bladder after death.

Morgagni entertains the same opinion with regard to the effects of a syphilitic taint.

Scarpa, a high authority on these subjects, thinks, " that even aneurism of the " aorta is much more frequently produced " by a slow morbid degeneration of it, " than by violent exertions of the whole " body, blows, or an increased impulse of " the heart.

" He adds, that the artery is nourished " and increased in the same manner as all " the other parts of the body ; it is vascu- " lar and organized, and therefore must " admit of the diseases to which vascular " and organized parts are liable ; and that " it is a fact, of which no doubt can be " entertained, that the proper coats of the " aorta are subject, from a slow internal " cause, to an ulcerated and steatomatous " disorganization, as well as a squamous " and earthy rigidity and brittleness. The " former of these he considers as mostly " connected with lues venerea.

" Both of these morbid states commence, " he thinks, in the inner membrane, or im- " mediately under it. At first, the surface

D D

" loses its beautiful smoothness, and be-
" comes irregular and wrinkled. It is after-
" wards interspersed with yellow spots,
" which are converted into grains and
" earthy scales, or into steatomatous and
" cheese-like concretions, which render the
" internal coat very brittle, and so slightly
" connected to the muscular, that upon be-
" ing merely scratched with a knife, or the
" point of a nail, pieces are readily detach-
" ed from it ; and on being cut, it gives a
" crackling sound, similar to the breaking
" of the shell of an egg. This ossification
" cannot be said to be proper to old age,
" since it is sometimes met with in patients
" not much advanced in life. In most
" cases the canal is constricted ; in the
" highest degree we find true ulceration,
" and at last aneurism in all stages."

It may be added, that the symptoms of
this change are often so obscure, as to give
very uncertain evidence of its existence in
the living body. We wonder sometimes at
the extensive havock that has been produced with so little warning. Morgagni, in a man who died suddenly from
rupture of the aorta, and whose case I

am surprised not to see quoted with
other examples of diseased coronaries,
found the aorta and its branches covered internally with prominencies and
pustules, which extended especially into
the subclavians, carotids, and coronaries;
one of the coronaries was besides dilated to nearly the size of the left ca-
rotid; the coats were easily separable
from each other, and the prominencies
contained a pulpy matter; and yet this
patient had no symptoms referrible to
such a cause, but some emaciation for
the last two or three years, and for the
same period an occasional feeling like
that of an approaching deliquium; *inter-
no quodam sensu, ac si deficeret.** In
others on the contrary, there is reason
to observe, that the very first rudiments
of ossification are marked by considerable sufferings. Whether it is, that in
such instances the disease is less confined to the internal membrane, or that
there is superadded a stricture from some
constitutional cause, the action of the

* Morgagni Epistolæ, xxvii. Artic. 28.

parts is greatly impeded, and they are incapable of that dilatation and contraction required on great exertions, in consequence of which arise pain and the signs of obstructed circulation. Nor is it so extraordinary that these effects should be produced in some, as it is unaccountable that they should be absent in any.

This slow ossific process, much more the active one superadded to it, may probably in its early stages be sometimes removed by proper treatment, or by the efforts of nature; the parts may as yet be but little altered in their structure; and that little, time may perhaps in some degree correct. It is possible that the patient may pass a long life without the recurrence of such symptoms. But it is more than probable, that irregularities, exertion, cold, suppression of gout, or the drying up of drains, will some time or other bring them back, and with them a gradual but finally very decided change in the structure, as well as functions, of the suffering organ. It becomes unable to support the circulation through the common accidents and

12

exertions of life. The fit comes on from the slightest movement, and even in that necessary pause from exertion which sleep occasions. *. Nor is it to be wondered at, that the neighbouring parts should in some degree suffer, that there should be su-, perficial marks of inflammation on the membranes, water accumulated in the chest or pericardium, and what has appeared to me to occur in an unusual proportion, adhesions of the lungs to the pleura on the left side, and very near the heart.

In the paroxysm, it is hardly possible that they should be quiescent, amidst the distress of that vital organ. The heart itself has been known to retain a palpitating motion, though the pulse disappeared at the wrist. The stomach sympathizes, sometimes the bladder. There are often signs of an affection of the diaphragm, of the other muscles of the tho-

* It is worthy of remark, that in two cases, I. and IV. this nightly distress, and a desire to fly to the open window for relief, came on amongst the first symptoms, and gradually disappeared as the disorder advanced.

rax, the pectoralis major which passes to the left arm, and even the deltoid. That this propagated pain is a muscular as well as a nervous sympathy, there is every reason to believe, both from the parts where it sometimes terminates, and from an affection decidedly muscular, which I have observed in one instance of this disease, and in several of rheumatism or gout suddenly attacking the heart. The muscles connecting the arm to the chest were not only painful, but their small fibres were affected with a twitching and vellication remarkably noticed by the patients, and in some degree visible to the observer.

Whatever difference of opinion may still subsist as to the constitutional cause, which brings on changes of structure in the arterial system generally, and the particular varieties of those changes, it is undeniable, that gouty and rheumatic habits are most subject to the angina pectoris; but whether it is that ossifications near the heart occur more frequently in such habits, or that a slighter degree of them produces a great impression, may admit of doubt. This disorder makes a slow progress with indolent, rich, gouty, persons; but I have seen it most rapidly destructive, in a spare rheumatic habit, subject not indeed to the acute form of rheumatism, but to nightly pains without swelling. Particularly, if under these circumstances the patient is still obliged to encounter manual labour and hard living, he cannot last many months.

It is remarkable, that the subjects of the angina pectoris are almost exclusively of the male sex.

The treatment of this disease is very undetermined and inefficient; nor can it be otherwise whilst so many symptoms obviously spasmodic are mixed with mal-organization, and the commencement and even nature of this latter are not agreed on.

Where the habit is gouty, every thing that will drive that disorder to the extremities, a most arduous attempt, is advis-

able ; and what will correct the disposition
to it ; for which purpose, soda and magnesia, I believe, answer best.

If the cause is rheumatic, it is still more
difficult to correct that distemper, or even
to transfer it to the surface.

In all, rest both of body and mind is to
be enjoined, with drains, and a moderately
relaxed state of the bowels.

The diet must vary with the general
health of the subject, but should, I think,
be as temperate, as that will admit. In the
aneurismal diathesis, abstinence to a great
extent has been recommended by Valsalva,
Guattani, and others, and by Dr. Fothergill in the angina pectoris, to remove a
supposed cause of it, an accumulation of
fat about the heart. Dr. Heberden, however, who had much experience in those
cases, and whose opinion is entitled to
great weight, thinks that a generous diet is
proper, and that we should not look for
the cure in those plans which lower the
strength. In determining this point, the
cause of the attack should be duly considered. Gout can rarely be driven to the

surface by a very low diet, but at the same
time admits of great caution in the choice
of food, and is benefited by it.   It is, however, hardly necessary to enlarge on that
point here.   Rheumatism is more inflammatory, and may seem to call for great
abstinence, particularly with regard to wine;
but that it ever will be removed from its
seat in the chest by this plan, I can by no
means assert.   Something, perhaps, may
be thus done, towards suspending the
progress of the disease.   Where the symptoms depend on neither of these acrimo-
nies, but on an original affection of the
parts, or external violence, as in Case V.,
an unusual moderation in diet may probably be adopted with advantage, as recommended for aneurism by the authors
quoted above.

Issues in the thighs have been partially
successful.   It may be some encouragement to add, that a gentleman, who had
never for a single week been free from the
disease for ten years together, lost every
vestige of it for the last nine months
of his life, during which he suffered from
ulcers of the lower extremities.   The sur-

face of the chest, opposite the heart, has been sometimes recommended for such a drain. I have not found experience to justify the hopes entertained. The inflammation excited by the caustic appeared to me in one instance, to irritate, and bring on the paroxysm. And the superior advantage of irritations in the lower extremities is strongly confirmed by the following case :

A. B., who had had one attack of the gout, about twenty years before, was recommended by me to open an issue in the region of the heart, on account of fits of the Angina Pectoris, exquisitely marked. During the forming and separation of the sloughs, the paroxysms greatly increased, and placed him in extreme danger. In this urgent state, mustard cataplasms, quickened with oil of turpentine, were applied to the feet ; and in ten minutes he was perfectly relieved. His unwillingness to bear pain induced him then to remove them. The distressing sensations on his chest quickly returned, and he was obliged to submit to a renewal of the cataplasms, which again operated almost

as a charm. An imperfect gout continued in the great toe for some weeks,
and for a long time after he had a true
sciatica.

Against an issue in the left arm, the
same objections do not hold, as against
those on the chest; and it may be added
in favour of it, that it has proved very serviceable in some severe affections of the
heart.

In the paroxysm, little has generally been
attempted. But when we recollect how
much of spasm mixes itself with the attack,
and that, perhaps, even the heart and aorta
are in some cases affected in that manner,
as is rendered particularly probable by the
dissection in Dr. Heberden's case, opiates
may be thought likely to render service.
Dr. Hunt of Dartmouth taught me the
safety of such a practice, who in a case of
this kind, in which we were consulted together, gave on the emergency, before my
arrival, ninety drops of tincture of opium.
The patient alluded to had experienced
many attacks of the angina pectoris; on
this occasion it was provoked by some very
slight bodily exertion; and he had remain-

ed for a long time in an entire deliquium, as far as the circulation was concerned, but a full possession of the faculties of the mind ; an awful state, hardly belonging to this world, and which whoever witnesses can never forget. *   The tincture of opium in divided doses soon began to relieve him ; and when I arrived about an hour after, the pulse had recovered some strength, and the pain and angor cordis were removed.   I have imitated this practice in other cases, but not with entire success.   It appears, however, to be safe, and where the habit is gouty, to be very beneficial.   Tincture of opium is likewise used with advantage, as Dr. Heberden informs us, to prevent the attack at night.

A tea-spoonful of æther has now and then carried off the paroxysm.

We may add, as a remedy worthy the trial, the immersion of the affected arm in water, as hot as can be borne.   I have

---

* The late Mr. John Hunter suffered such a paroxysm, in which the pulse at the wrist ceased for three quarters of an hour, and he found himself at times not breathing ; yet sensation and the voluntary actions were perfect. — See Home's Life of Hunter, page 46.

used it on Morgagni's authority, and found great relief from it in some anomalous complaints of the heart, where the left arm was painful.

From what has been advanced, page 410, it is obvious, that rubefacients to the lower extremities, should not be omitted, particularly where gout is suspected. A respectable practitioner in this county, obtained relief for many years by that application; one night he asked for them, as he often had done, but before they could be prepared, he had breathed his last. In another instance they had been used with advantage; but on the fatal attack, they failed to produce any pain or inflammation, though applied repeatedly, and of great strength; and the patient lingered for many hours, sensible, but without a pulse.

It has been already remarked, that the paroxysm of the angina pectoris partakes generally of the character of a deliquium; and on that account, it has received from Dr. Parry the appropriate name of syncope anginosa. Are there any cases to which that term is not applicable, in consequence of the pulse remaining unaltered? I leave it to those who have seen the disease in a slighter form than I have done, to determine this point. Dr. Heberden undoubtedly had such cases in his view, since he says, that the pulse is at least sometimes not disturbed by this pain, and consequently the heart is not affected by it.

It appears, likewise, that causes seated in the abdomen may produce symptoms having a character of great resemblance to the disease above-described. Dr. Percival's case renders this probable. It has occurred to me to see three instances of the same kind. The persons alluded to, besides having a sallow complexion, pain of the epigastric region, bilious or clay-coloured discharges, &c., were likewise subject, on exercise, but particularly after loading the stomach, to a straitness of the lower part of the sternum, palpitations, excessive anxiety about the heart, pain stretching thence to the mammæ and both arms, and a quick hurried pulse. Bleeding gave temporary relief; but opiates were extremely injurious. Two of these persons died with signs of a schirrous liver; a third was cured by calomel, and now, twelve years after, enjoys robust health, and is capable of much exertion. Such patients greatly want evacuations by mercury, and cannot bear the least restraint of the bowels. I remarked in these an increase of the circulation; but many adventitious causes, or even the greater intensity of the original cause, may, I believe, convert palpitations into deliquia; and we shall then be greatly deceived in our conclusions, unless we take other circumstances into the account.

After all that can be done on such subjects, we shall, I fear, ever have to lament the difficulty of applying to particular cases those rules which are so precisely laid down by authors. Every case has some peculiarities. Nosology treats of genera and species; nature gives us individuals; and in these we meet varieties and combinations both of local and constitutional disease, which frequently embarrass the most accurate observer, and set all arrangement at defiance.

THE END.

Printed by A. Strahan,
Printers-Street, London.

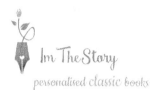

Im The Story
personalised classic books

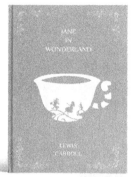

"Beautiful gift.. lovely finish.
My Niece loves it, so precious!"

Helen R Brumfield

⭐⭐⭐⭐⭐

UNIQUE GIFT

FOR KIDS, PARTNERS
AND FRIENDS

Timeless books such as:

Kids

Alice in Wonderland · The Jungle Book · The Wonderful Wizard of Oz
Peter and Wendy · Robin Hood · The Prince and The Pauper
The Railway Children · Treasure Island · A Christmas Carol

Adults

Romeo and Juliet · Dracula

Highly Customizable

Change Books Title

Replace Characters Names with yours

Upload Photo for inside page

Add Inscriptions

Visit
Im The Story .com
and order yours today!

CPSIA information can be obtained
at www.ICGtesting.com
Printed in the USA
BVHW090859280819
556854BV00004B/821/P